CHANGING EATING AND EXERCISE BEHAVIOUR

CHANGING EATING AND EXERCISE BEHAVIOUR

PAULA HUNT

and

MELVYN HILLSDON

**Blackwell
Science**

© 1996 by Paula Hunt and Melvyn Hillsdon
Blackwell Science Ltd
Editorial Offices:
Osney Mead, Oxford OX2 0EL
25 John Street, London WC1N 2BL
23 Ainslie Place, Edinburgh EH3 6AJ
238 Main Street, Cambridge
    Massachusetts 02142, USA
54 University Street, Carlton
    Victoria 3053, Australia

Other Editorial Offices:
Arnette Blackwell SA
    224, Boulevard Saint Germain
    75007 Paris, France

Blackwell Wissenschafts-Verlag GmbH
    Kurfürstendamm 57
    10707 Berlin, Germany

    Zehetnergasse 6
    A-1140 Wien
    Austria

First published 1996

Set in 10 on 12.5 pt Century Book
by DP Photosetting, Aylesbury, Bucks
Printed and bound in Great Britain by
Hartnolls Ltd, Bodmin, Cornwall

The Blackwell Science logo is a trade
mark of Blackwell Science Ltd,
registered at the United Kingdom
Trade Mark Registry

DISTRIBUTORS

Marston Book Services Ltd
PO Box 269
Abingdon
Oxon OX14 4YN
(Orders: Tel: 01235 465500
        Fax: 01235 465555)

USA
Blackwell Science, Inc.
238 Main Street
Cambridge, MA 02142
(*Orders:* Tel: 800 215-1000
          617 876-7000
      Fax: 617 492-5263)

Canada
Copp Clark, Ltd
2775 Matheson Blvd East
Mississauga, Ontario
Canada, L4W 4P7
(*Orders:* Tel: 800 263-4374
          905 238-6074)

Australia
Blackwell Science Pty Ltd
54 University Street
Carlton, Victoria 3053
(*Orders:* Tel: 03 9347 0300
          Fax: 03 9349 3016)

A catalogue record for this title
is available from the British Library

ISBN 0–632–03927–2

Library of Congress
Cataloging-in-Publication Data

Hunt, Paula, SRD.
    Changing eating and exercise
behaviour/Paula Hunt and Melvyn
Hillsdon.
        p.   cm.
    Includes bibliographical references
and index.
    ISBN 0–632–03927–2 (pb)
    1. Weight loss–Psychological aspects.
2. Exercise–Psychological aspects.
3. Health behavior.   4. Food habits.
5. Client-centred psychotherapy.
6. Health counseling.   7. Nutrition
counseling.   I. Hillsdon, Melvyn.
II. Title.
RM222.2.H858   1996
613.7–dc20   96-16809
                                     CIP

Dedication
I dedicate this book to the memory of my father, Anthony Melville
Hillsdon, a great friend and role model.

Melvyn Hillsdon

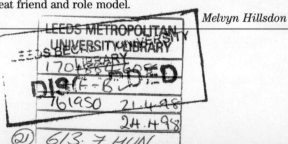

Contents

Preface

We are constantly being asked for help from professionals on how they can be more successful in 'making' their patients or clients adopt and maintain a healthy lifestyle. Giving them accurate and up-to-date advice on how they should change, in a professional and well-informed manner is, apparently, just not working. Between us we have run many training sessions on skills development for professionals working in the diet and fitness fields. It has become clear, based on our own difficulties with clients, from our training experiences and from our reading of the scientific literature, that information alone is not enough and that if professionals believe that their mission is to *make* people change, they will usually fail.

Hence, in this book our emphasis is on a client-centred approach. It is clear from the scientific literature that being client-centred is fundamental for effective interventions. There is also an irrefutable picture of the exact nature of the core qualities and skills which are highly desirable for a helping relationship. What else is important is much less clear. The evidence is not complete and in some cases scanty, simply because the research has not yet been done. We are confident, however, that many of the findings from research into other health behaviours and counselling approaches will apply in varying degrees to diet and exercise. We are especially convinced where studies replicated in the different behavioural and lifestyle areas show a consistent picture. The literature on which this book is based is detailed fully in the reference list.

We have borrowed aspects of different counselling styles and techniques for the helping process described in this book. Examples include motivational interviewing and some of the cognitive behavioural approaches. We are cautious, however, in suggesting that this book is based on complete or robust science or that our

approaches can sweepingly be adopted as evidence-based practice. It is a combination of evidence and clinical experience. We
look forward to seeing further published research into effective
interventions for diet and exercise.

Helping clients with behaviour change is perhaps less a
mechanical science and more an art. It is fluid and dynamic. You
never know exactly how your client will respond, what she or he
will say next, nor what path the consultation will take. You will
need, therefore, to have a medley of different responses at your
finger tips and be prepared to allow the consultation to flow, whilst
keeping a grip on where, ultimately, it is heading. The counsellor's
role is to keep track of the general theme and to orchestrate, whilst
listening and responding intuitively to the client's concerns and
actions. All of this has to be done in the time constraints within
which you work.

The risk of teaching a theoretical framework from which to
work, as we have done in this book, is that the art is lost and the
approach to helping people change their behaviour becomes
mechanistic and rigid. We urge readers to recognise that the sec-
tioning of the different components of change within this book are
merely for convenience, both yours and ours! Different aspects of
change are featured, accompanied by the relevant mode of intervention. Appropriate techniques and styles of questioning, listening, responding and information giving are suggested at each stage.
In reality, however, helping clients through the course of change
will often not be quite so logical. There is much overlap between
the stages of change described in the book. And it may take time; a
set of brief consultations over a period of several months is more
likely to be effective than a longer one-off session at the start.

This text has been designed with easy access for the reader in
mind. Some issues are generic and apply similarly to diet and
exercise and so have been dealt with as such. Examples given to
illustrate such points may be about general lifestyle change, just
eating, just exercise, or a bit of both. Other parts of the book are
more specific to the field of eating and exercise and have been dealt
with separately, with examples of both where it seems helpful.

Where we have used case scenarios and/or given examples of
dialogue the cases are realistic but fictitious. We have attempted to
use gender in a random and non-stereotyping way and have used
'he' and 'she' interchangeably throughout the text when describing
clients in the third person.

A book like this does not happen without a lot of help from others. We are indebted to colleagues, mentors and friends who have been generous with their time and ideas. In particular, thanks to Gill Cowburn for her invaluable comments on an earlier draft. We are also grateful to our partners, Tim and Jane, for their relentless support – both emotional and practical – throughout the creation of this book.

We hope this handbook gives insight, a little more confidence and a ray of hope to those of you who feel frustrated with your current efforts to help clients eat more healthily or become more active.

Paula Hunt
Melvyn Hillsdon

Part One
Theory

Chapter 1
A Role for Professionals

Primary care and fitness professionals are uniquely placed to help change peoples' diet and exercise habits. Primary health care teams have access to the population; almost 80% of people visit their doctor's surgery at least once in one year (Royal College of General Practitioners 1995). Many people are registered with the same practice for most of their life, giving health professionals continued access over many years. This is especially valuable for giving repeated and continuous care and support regarding life-style change. In addition, health professionals are repeatedly reported as one of the most trusted sources of food and health advice (McCluney 1988, National Dairy Council 1992), suggesting that they are perceived as highly credible in this role, and are the general public's preferred source of information and support on health issues.

Primary care teams are charged to work in a variety of ways to promote the health of the practice population, particularly now that the Government's health promotion package reimburses general practice for a range of different activities rather than clinic sessions only. Indeed, the role of primary care professionals as health promoters is increasingly important as the British National Health Service changes its structure and role. The reforms of the early 1990s have resulted in a primary care-led health care system that places much greater emphasis on health promotion and disease prevention than ever before. The days are gone when the health service only treated the sick and had no vision for preventing ill-health.

For health professionals to realise their full potential as agents for lifestyle change, they will have to update their knowledge and acquire new skills. They are often frustrated by their inability to help clients achieve long-term dietary change or to take more exercise on a regular and permanent basis. Being equipped with the new approaches described in this book is more likely to lead to beneficial changes resulting in improved health and well-being, which will be more rewarding both for the health professionals and for their clients.

A dual strategy for helping people change to a healthier lifestyle is thought to be the most favourable. That is, combining a secondary prevention approach, targeting those at high risk of chronic disease, with a broader primary prevention programme aimed at the whole population.

Possible approaches, therefore, for helping people change eating and exercise behaviour in the primary care setting include:

- individual advice-giving, with a leaflet;
- individual counselling and support;
- group counselling and support;
- campaigns and displays within the health centre; and
- community-based activities outside the health centre.

The first three listed will tend to be secondary prevention activities, targeted at those who have been identified, through screening, as being at risk of disease. The last two on the list are more likely to be primary prevention interventions, aiming to influence the whole of a population with blanket health promotion techniques, rather then filtering out those who would most benefit, in health terms, from change. This does not preclude individual or group approaches for primary prevention work; people may choose to attend one-to-one or group advice sessions out of general interest in health, rather than because they are at risk in any way.

Traditionally most of the health promotion work done by primary health care professionals, especially practice nurses and general practitioners, has involved consultations with individual patients on a one-to-one basis for brief advice or, time permitting, more thorough counselling and support. Little group work has been done, though in some instances community nurses, especially health visitors, have used this approach if a suitable room is available within the practice.

Few primary prevention activities, especially anything outside the health centre or surgery, have been tackled by primary health care professionals. With funding opportunities increasing, especially for developmental work which is to be evaluated, such projects may become more commonplace in the future.

It may be that primary prevention is best done in an environment which has less of a medical focus and is more closely associated with lifestyle change and wellness. An obvious place for this is in a health club or leisure centre. The role of the fitness professional as a health promoter thus becomes equally important to that of health professionals. People visiting sports and leisure facilities may be especially well motivated to adopt a healthy lifestyle, regardless of their risk, known or unknown, of chronic disease. Whatever their level of motivation, they will probably still need support. Seizing the opportunity to advise and support them should be seen as an important role for fitness professionals and should complement the service offered by health professionals.

To retain credibility, fitness professionals should make it their business to keep updated on health issues and to develop the special counselling skills described in this book. Being able to communicate clearly and constructively with clients whilst still showing empathy is a sophisticated skill which requires practice. Identifying barriers to change and helping people work with their own difficulties is challenging but highly rewarding. Regularly checking and supporting clients who have successfully made and sustained changes will be good for business too as a permanent commitment to exercising means continued use of the facilities!

Whilst the opportunities for one-to-one counselling on eating and exercise in the primary care setting are clear, there are some difficulties and limitations. The most commonly mentioned is that of lack of time. There is no doubt that giving effective support to individuals can be time-consuming. The approaches described in this book, however, recognise this constraint and suggest ways to make the consultations as brief as possible whilst still having an impact. Combining brevity with effectiveness means listening carefully and asking exactly the right questions, at exactly the right time. This is discussed more fully in Part Two.

The constraints caused by health professionals' poor knowledge and limited skills when giving diet and exercise advice are widely documented (Wallace & Haines 1988, Francis *et al.* 1989, Baron *et al.* 1990, Murray *et al.* 1992, Cade & O'Connell 1993). Whilst this book aims to address this in part, it is essential that professionals seek appropriate training to enable them to develop and practise the skills outlined. Simply reading the book will not suffice! In addition, there is an onus on all professionals to keep updated on the technical aspects of nutrition, sport and exercise. Although the authors are confident that the advice in this book is accurate at the time of writing, the growing research base in both of these fields means that the picture is evolving rapidly. Policy and practice will undoubtedly change in response to published research findings and the credibility of professionals will be affected if they do not keep abreast of modern thinking.

It is clear from studies that the need for consistent advice is also key; the public commonly report that it seems the experts are always changing their minds, especially with respect to dietary advice, and they cite this as a major barrier to change (Sheiham *et al.*, 1990). Not only the message but the messenger too must be accurate, clear and consistent. The identification of and access to local specialists who can offer training courses or telephone advice and updates via newsletters and circulars is invaluable. For nutrition and dietary information, state registered dietitians are available via the local health promotion unit or hospital. Independent authoritative bodies, such as the Health Education Authority, have resources on healthy eating. Specialist advice about sports and exercise is available from the Exercise Association for England, or more locally from the council's leisure services department.

A further limitation for many professionals when carrying out lifestyle interventions in primary care is the possible lack of support from management, the employing organisation or from immediate colleagues. There is some scepticism amongst those who are unconvinced of the value of doing this type of work in primary care. Some would argue that the cost-effectiveness is questionable or that the limited evidence to date about effectiveness *per se*, does not make the task worthwhile.

Although this field is relatively under-researched at present, there is some published evidence that one-to-one interventions by professionals can be effective and these are discussed more fully (by the British Family Heart Study Group 1994, ICRF OXCHECK Study Group 1994). What is important is that people are clear about the extent of the contribution that one-to-one interventions for lifestyle change can be expected to make. The impact should not be overestimated and change is unlikely if such interventions are not supported by a range of societal, structural and organisational changes which make healthy choices easier for individuals. In isolation from such public health policy changes, one-to-one

counselling is probably of fairly limited value. With the right supporting conditions, however, its contribution can be of great significance. Helping people change eating and exercise behaviour
can be a highly rewarding and important role for health and fitness
professionals.

Chapter 2
The Case for Change

Why change?

There are undoubted health benefits of eating a well-balanced diet and taking regular exercise. Diet and physical activity are two of many things which can affect the risk of common diseases, including coronary heart disease (CHD), strokes and some cancers. Other risk factors include family history, smoking, stress, excess body weight, high blood pressure and high blood cholesterol level. The more of these risk factors which apply, the greater a person's own risk of developing diseases which can greatly reduce quality of life and cause premature death. The Government's strategy for health, *The Health of the Nation*, has identified the need to change peoples' eating and exercise habits in order to prevent disease and meet its targets for good health by the year 2005 (Department of Health 1992).

Changing diet and exercise behaviour is a positive step which does not only reduce long-term risk of disease; it may have many short- and medium-term benefits too. People have reported immediate benefits of changing to a healthier lifestyle, including having more energy, feeling more relaxed, sleeping better, feeling more self-confident and generally having a greater sense of well-being.

Medium-term benefits may include a range of things such as suffering less from ailments like constipation or headaches, being part of a new and supportive social group or feeling more comfortable in clothes that were once tight. The benefits to overall health are much more long-term and sometimes less obvious to individuals. There is no doubt, however, that a more active and healthy lifestyle will put people at lower risk of diseases such as CHD, strokes and some cancers, as well as reducing their risk of developing diabetes in later life. It will also reduce the risk of becoming obese which, in its own right, is linked with many debilitating conditions including back pain, breathing problems, arthritis (especially in the hips and knees), painful feet, gallstones, high blood pressure and heartburn.

The case for eating

Despite what the lay press would seem to suggest, there is now unequivocal evidence from the scientific literature about the need for population-wide dietary change. Cohort studies, epidemiological evidence and clinical research trials demonstrate clearly and consistently that changes in risk factors through dietary means can have an influence on the course of disease (e.g. CHD, stroke, some cancers and diabetes). Many studies have shown a positive effect of dietary intervention by using biochemical and clinical outcome measures, such as reduced blood cholesterol levels, reduced blood pressure and reduced body weight. Benefits have been shown by a variety of research groups doing dietary intervention studies on hypercholesterolaemic patients (Dallongville 1994, Denke & Grundy 1994, McGowan *et al.* 1994) and on people who are overweight or obese (Geppert & Splett 1991, Cousins *et al.* 1992). Other studies have assessed the extent of dietary change achieved and linked this with positive changes in blood measurements and body weight (Beresford 1992, Keuhl 1993).

Following several years of uncertainty there is now strong evidence for a causal relationship between sodium consumption and blood pressure which has been agreed and accepted by scientists and doctors (Department of Health 1994a). An average reduction of 50 mmol sodium (current intakes of sodium are about 170 mmol/day in men and 130 mmol/day in women) per day (3 g salt per day) has been estimated to result in an average reduction in systolic blood pressure of about 3.5 mmHg. This effect would be greater with longer-term change, as the rise of blood pressure with age would also be reduced.

A review involving a meta-analysis by Truswell (1994) provides strong and unequivocal evidence that dietary counselling is effective in terms of the ultimate outcome measure (health gain) indicated by reduced mortality and morbidity. He showed that overall the total death rate was 6% less and there were 13% fewer coronary events in intervention groups compared with control groups in 17 randomised control trials for dietary intervention. Another study has shown that a 10% lowering of plasma cholesterol, which can be achieved through moderate dietary change, is associated with a 50% reduction in CHD risk at 40 years and a 20% reduction in risk at 70 years (Law *et al.* 1994). There is no doubt that giving dietary advice can improve health.

The complex interrelationship between food, nutrients, risk factors and disease is summarised in Figure 2.1. A bonus of changing to a healthier diet is that the same changes have a positive effect on the risk of many different diseases, so multiple advantages are accrued. For example, the risk of cancer, CHD and stroke is reduced by exactly the same dietary means.

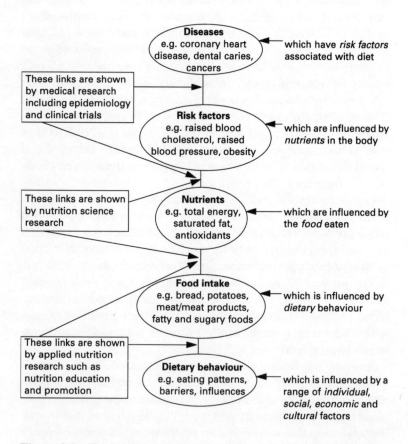

Figure 2.1   The link between food, nutrients, risk factors and disease.

The case for physical activity

The case for physical activity is as strong as that for dietary change but to date, despite the abundance of American publications, there are few official UK reports making specific policy recommendations about exercise for the general public. Observational evidence demonstrates that being physically active and fit reduces the risk of developing coronary heart disease, at least in men. Recent reviews have concluded that people who are more physically active and physically fit are at a lower risk for CHD (Powell *et al.* 1987). A meta-analysis of physical activity in the prevention of coronary heart disease concluded that the relative risk of developing CHD in the least active compared to the most active was 1.9 (Berlin & Colditz 1990). This means that the most active subjects are about half as likely to die from cardiovascular disease as the least active subjects . While there is no direct experimental evidence for the effect of physical activity on the primary prevention of CHD, extensive observational data support the conclusion that physical activity and physical fitness are inversely associated with the incidence of CHD.

Though the relative risk of CHD associated with inactivity is similar in magnitude to other risk factors such as smoking, hypertension and elevated serum cholesterol (Pooling Project Research Group 1978), the prevalence of physical inactivity is considerably greater (Figure 2.2). The Allied Dunbar National Fitness Survey estimated that 'around 70% or more of each age group were below an acceptable activity level threshold that would confer significant health and functional benefits' (Allied Dunbar 1992).

Theoretically, such figures suggest that removing physical inactivity as a risk factor in a population would have a greater preventive effect on future CHD incidence than eliminating smoking, elevated serum cholesterol or hypertension. Apart from its role in reducing the risk of CHD, physical activity appears to be beneficial in reducing the risk of stroke, hypertension, non-insulin dependent diabetes, osteoporosis, depression and some cancers (Bouchard *et al.* 1994). Not only can physical activity itself reduce the risk of the development of CHD directly, but it can be an integral part of the management of other risk factors. For example, regular endurance exercise lowers both systolic and diastolic blood pressure by approximately 10 mmHg (Fagard & Tipton

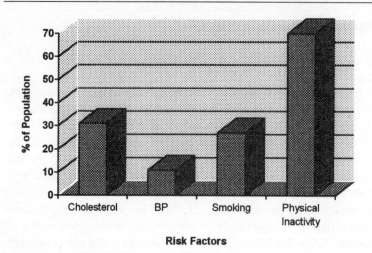

Risk Factors

Figure 2.2   Prevalence of major risk factors for cardiovascular disease (data taken from the Health Survey for England (1995) and Allied Dunbar (1992)).

1994). People who are more physically active also tend to have a more favourable blood lipid profile than those who are less active (Stefanick & Wood 1994).

Physical activity can provide important health benefits for those with chronic conditions as well as the apparently healthy. Conditions such as arthritis, chronic obstructive pulmonary disease, diabetes, osteoporosis, depression, low back pain and cardiovascular disease show positive changes as a result of a programme of regular moderate intensity exercise (Bouchard et al. 1994).

The role of physical activity in the rehabilitation of patients with coronary heart disease is receiving increasing attention. Meta-analyses of randomised controlled trials of the effect of cardiac rehabilitation programmes report a 20% reduction in total mortality, a 22% reduction in cardiovascular mortality and a 25% reduction in the risk of fatal reinfarction. In addition to these reductions in mortality, most patients engaging in cardiac rehabilitation report improved well-being and exercise tolerance and a reduction in anxiety (Quaglietti & Froelicher 1994).

The importance of physical activity in protecting, improving, maintaining and regaining one's health should not be underestimated. There is now sufficient evidence to support the promotion of regular physical activity in the majority of the inactive population.

What and how much to change?

Eating

In 1994 the Committee on Medical Aspects of Food Policy (COMA) report provided clear recommendations for nutritional and food-specific changes in the UK diet (Department of Health 1994a), which support conclusions of previous reports from the same committee in 1991 (Department of Health 1991) and 1984 (Department of Health 1984) and by the World Health Organisation in 1990 (World Health Organisation 1990). The recommendations have changed very little since the early 1980s, thereby reinforcing the strength of the scientifically based message and the need for all messengers to be telling the public the same story. Quantified nutrition targets have been set by the Government, by COMA and in the *Health of the Nation* strategy document. A summary of the COMA 1994 recommendations, specifically for reducing cardio-vascular disease through dietary means, is shown in Table 2.1. These complement the dietary targets, which are written in nutritional terms, highlighted in the *Health of the Nation* document (Department of Health 1992), and are as follows:

- Reducing the population average intake of *total fat* from 40% to 35% of energy by the year 2005 (a 12% reduction).
- Reducing the population average intake of *saturated fat* from 17% to 11% of energy by the year 2005 (a 35% reduction).
- Reducing the prevalence of *obesity* in the adult population (16–64 years olds) from 8% to 6% in men and from 12% to 8% in women by the year 2005 (a 25% reduction in men and a 33% reduction in women).

An implementation strategy for achieving these population targets has been set out in the *Eat Well* document produced by the Government's Nutrition Task Force (Department of Health 1994b). So, how likely is it that the dietary changes required to meet these targets will be made? A large nutritional and dietary survey of British adults in 1990 (Gregory *et al.* 1990) showed that at that time 85% of the nationally representative sample were eating more fat as a proportion of their overall energy intake than the recommended level. In addition, 45% of adult men and 35% of adult women were either overweight or obese. Although the National Food Survey (Office of Population and Census Surveys 1994) shows small

Table 2.1 Recommendations for reducing cardiovascular disease risk through dietary means. From the Committee on Medical Aspects of Food Policy (COMA) 1994.

Nutritional issue	Food	Recommendation for change
Body weight	Amount and balance of all foods.	People should maintain a desirable body weight (BMI 20–25) as they get older through regular physical activity and eating appropriate amounts of food conforming to the dietary patterns below.
Saturated fat	Dairy and meat products, fat spreads.	Reduce average contribution of saturated fatty acids to dietary energy to no more than 10%.
n-6 polyunsaturated fat	Oils and polyunsaturated margarines.	No further increase.
n-3 long chain polyunsaturated fat	Oily fish.	Increase population average consumption from 0.1 g to 0.2 g per day (1.5 g per week).
Trans fatty acids	Hydrogenated fat in margarines and shortenings and products made from them, e.g. biscuits, pastries; also dairy and meat products.	No increase in current average of 2% dietary energy.
Monounsaturates	In many foods.	No specific recommendation.
Total fat	In many foods.	Reduce average contribution of total fat to dietary energy to about 35%.
Dietary cholesterol	Eggs, shellfish, offal.	Present intake should not rise.
Sodium	Common salt – at the table, in cooking and in processed foods.	Reduce average intake of sodium in adults from current 150 mmol/day (9 g salt) to 100 mmol/day (6 g salt).
Potassium	Potatoes, other vegetables, fruit, meat and milk.	Increase average intake of potassium in adults to about 3.5 g/day (90 mmol/day).
Carbohydrates	Potatoes, bread, pasta, rice, breakfast cereals, (sugars*).	Increase proportion of energy derived from carbohydrate to approx. 50% to restore the energy deficit following a reduction in the dietary intake of fat.

* Although an increased intake of carbohydrate is recommended, of which sugar is an example, high intakes of sugars can have undesirable effects on dental health, and in the obese can predispose to undesirable metabolic effects.

encouraging changes in the types of food eaten, these are modest. They include for example, more low fat milks being consumed, and slightly more fish, fruit, potatoes and bread, and marginally less confectionery and biscuits. However, the rising prevalence of obesity may indicate that much greater changes are required, especially in the amounts of certain foods consumed and the amount of exercise taken.

In addition, the above data should be interpreted with caution. Although they give a good picture of what people eat at home, until recently they excluded any food eaten outside the home, which now accounts for about a third of people's energy intake (Loughridge 1991, Adamson 1995). It is likely that the foods absent from the National Food Survey data are confectionery, crisps and high-fat fast foods.

The small changes in the range and proportion of different foods eaten have made a minimal contribution to improving the nutritional profile of the population. Although there has been a small reduction in average saturated fat intake, energy from total fat has barely fallen at all and the prevalence of obesity is actually increasing, so moving away from, rather than towards the target.

The possible nature and extent of food-specific changes required to meet the nutritional targets in the average UK diet across the adult population have been estimated (Bingham 1991). These estimates relate to achieving a population average so will not necessarily apply to every individual. Bingham's projection includes doubling vegetable and bread intake, eating half as much again of fruit and potatoes, halving current consumption of biscuits, cakes, puddings, chips, crisps, other high fat/fried products, chocolate, sugar, preserves and sugary drinks, and switching from whole to semi-skimmed milk, from saturated to low fat spreads and to leaner cuts of meats. She notes that the political acceptance of the potential for good health through food represents a remarkable change of emphasis that should have wide ranging consequences for agriculture, the food industry, advertising, food science, departments of public health, and ultimately the consumer. Achieving these targets, however, is not going to be easy.

Subsequently, the COMA report (Department of Health 1994a) has made positive food recommendations to the population which include:

- eating two portions of fish weekly, of which one should be oily fish;
- using reduced fat spreads and dairy products instead of full fat products;
- replacing fats high in saturated fatty acids (e.g. butter, fully hydrogenated margarine, lard, ghee) with oils/fats which are low in saturated fatty acids and rich in monounsaturates (e.g. low fat spreads, rapeseed oil, olive oil);
- eating 50% more vegetables;
- eating 50% more fruit;
- eating 50% more bread; and
- eating 50% more potatoes.

The report also discusses the implications for foods and diets more fully. It explains that for the recommendations to be achieved in the context of a nutritionally adequate diet there would have to be major changes in the national average pattern of food consumption in Britain. The diet would have to contain significantly less saturated and total fat and sodium and significantly more fruits and vegetables, complex carbohydrates, non-starch polysaccharides (or fibre) and potassium. It suggests that it seems likely that any changes in the national eating patterns would result from a variety of changes across the whole range of foodstuffs, rather than drastic changes in one or two. In addition to the specific changes already recommended, people would also have to consume less fatty meat and meat products, less high fat dairy food and fewer full fat spreading fats.

The requirement is for a reduction in national *per capita* average consumption of approximately 15 g of total fat and 11 g of saturated fat each day. Again, it is stressed that this applies to the population average and so does not necessarily apply to all individuals. Some examples of ways to achieve this are shown in Table 2.2.

The COMA report also includes a recommendation to reduce the average intake of common salt (sodium chloride) by the adult population from the current level of about 9 g per day (150 mmol/day) to about 6 g per day (100 mmol/day). Some examples of ways to achieve this are shown in Table 2.3.

Exercise

The amount of physical activity required to achieve the improvements to health indicated previously has been the cause of much

Table 2.2 Saving at least 15 g total fat and 11 g saturated fat in a day – some examples.

Food	Exchanged for:	Fat saving (g per portion)	Saturated fat saving (g per portion)
2 slices bread with butter	2 slices bread with low fat spread	11	9
Pie with 2 crusts	Pie with 1 crust	6	2
a. Total		*17*	*11*
Sponge cake with butter icing	Currant bun with low fat spread	11	3
Baked potato with butter	Baked potato with low fat spread	8	8
b. Total		*19*	*11*
1 bowl breakfast cereal with whole milk	1 bowl breakfast cereal with semi-skimmed milk	2	1
Baked potato with cheddar cheese	Baked potato with cottage cheese	16	10
c. Total		*18*	*11*
2 digestive biscuits	1 banana	7	3
Cheeseburger in a bun	Beefburger in a bun	5	3
1 thick and creamy yoghurt	1 low fat yoghurt	3	1
2 slices bread with butter	2 slices bread with polyunsaturated margarine	0	8
d. Total		*15*	*15*

debate. Is there a minimum amount of exercise that we need to do before we confer any benefit? Do we need to be active, fit or both? To be able to understand this debate it is important to be clear about what is meant by physical activity, exercise and physical fitness. Physical activity is normally described as 'any bodily

Table 2.3 Contributions to a saving of 2.5 g salt (or 1 g sodium) in a day – some examples.

Food	Exchange for:	Salt saving (g per portion)	Sodium saving (g per portion)
Peas boiled in salted water	Peas boiled in unsalted water	0.4	0.2
Spaghetti/rice boiled in salted water	Spaghetti/rice boiled in unsalted water	1.0	0.4
Salted peanuts (1 portion)	Fresh peanuts (unsalted) (1 portion)	0.5	0.2
Salted crisps (1 small packet)	Unsalted crisps (1 small packet)	0.7	0.3
Regular baked beans (1 portion)	Low salt baked beans (1 portion)	0.8	0.3
Stilton cheese (50 g)	Low fat cream cheese (50 g)	1.2	0.5
A bowl of high salt breakfast cereal, e.g. All Bran	A bowl of low salt breakfast cereal, e.g. Puffed Wheat, porridge oats	1.2	0.5
Adding salt to food at home (in cooking and at the table)	Not adding salt to food at home (in cooking and at the table)	1.5	0.6

movement produced by skeletal muscles that results in energy expenditure' and is normally measured in kilocalories per week (kcal/week). Exercise can be described as a form of physical activity that is 'planned, structured and repetitive bodily movement done to improve or maintain one or more components of physical fitness'. Physical fitness is 'a set of attributes that people have or achieve that relates to the ability to perform physical activity'.

Some of the early research into physical activity tended to support the 'threshold' argument for physical activity. That is, until a certain level of physical activity is achieved no significant benefits accrue. Current research, however, is frequently showing a 'dose-response' relationship to physical activity and CHD; that is, as physical activity increases the risk of CHD decreases. The amount of benefit derived from increased physical activity depends on the individual's initial physical activity level. Those people who are sedentary (taking no regular physical activity) would expect to gain most from increasing their physical activity. Those who already do some physical activity, however, are also likely to derive some additional health benefits from increasing their physical activity, as well as becoming physically fitter (Blair *et al.* 1992).

Physical fitness data show similar patterns to those on physical activity. Most studies again show an inverse relationship between mortality and physical fitness categories. That is, groups of people who are the most physically fit tend to live longer and *vice versa*. As with physical activity, a relatively small improvement in fitness in the least fit results in a relatively large reduction in mortality (Blair *et al.* 1989).

There is no doubt that sedentary living is one of the causes of CHD. Predicting the extent and type of activity required for optimum health, or defining an absolute desirable level of fitness is very difficult from existing data. The evidence is encouraging though, as it appears that substantial health benefits can be obtained from increased physical activity and fitness without the need to be vigorously active or incredibly fit. Important gains can be achieved by becoming moderately active and fit (Pate *et al.* 1995).

The current public health recommendation (USA) for physical activity is that every adult should accumulate 30 minutes or more of moderate intensity physical activity on most, preferably all, days of the week (Pate *et al.* 1995). The recommendation recognises the importance of moderate intensity physical activity and that physical activity can be accumulated in bouts as short as 10 minutes. The recommendation is equivalent to a daily 2 mile brisk walk. Being performed intermittently means that the target can be more easily incorporated into peoples' existing lifestyles by, for example, taking the stairs instead of the lift, getting off the bus a stop early, walking instead of driving short distances or cycling to and from work. This recommendation complements the earlier message to take at least 20 minutes of vigorous activity on no fewer than 3 days per week. The previous message was based on the health benefits to be achieved by improving physical fitness but it is now clear that less vigorous, but more prolonged, forms of physical activity are equally beneficial.

The recommendation is something to build up to. Those who are currently sedentary might start by including a few minutes walk each day, building up over a number of weeks and months. Any further reference to regular physical activity in this book will relate to these most recent recommendations. The terms physical activity and exercise will be used interchangeably.

When to change?

Not only why but when to change is a question people often consider. Many older adults imagine that irreversible damage has already been done and it is therefore too late to achieve any significant health benefits by changing their lifestyle now. Young adults may assume that they can lead an unhealthy lifestyle now and make amends later. Neither are completely true. The accumulative effect of unhealthy living over many years means that it is worth considering diet and exercise as early in life as possible. Conversely, although some harm may have resulted from many years of inactivity and poor diet, the effect can at least be halted and in some cases reversed if lifestyles change. It is never too late and although the research evidence is not yet clear, it has been suggested that people in their seventh and eighth decade can improve the quality of their lives and reduce their risk of ill health by adopting appropriate diet and exercise habits (Ahmed 1992).

Ideally everyone would eat healthily and exercise regularly as part of routine living, starting in early childhood and continuing into the later years. In reality, however, this is far from true. The data show that only 15–20% of adults in the UK have a healthy diet (Gregory *et al.* 1990, 1994) and 15–30% of adults take sufficient exercise for optimum health (Allied Dunbar, Sports Council 1992).

Chapter 3
Achieving Change

Effective approaches

Identifying and targeting those who are at risk of ill-health can be difficult and costly and a combination of approaches to promoting health is more likely to achieve the biggest overall benefit to the morbidity and mortality of a given population.

Primary prevention strategies, delivered *en mass* to a whole population or community, and involving no screening to identify those at risk of chronic disease, may have little effect on individuals *per se* but can make a meaningful impact on morbidity and mortality in the whole population. Conversely, secondary prevention, which is much more common in the primary health care setting, involves identifying people with risk factors or early symptoms of disease and offering intensive advice which will help delay the onset of or completely prevent the disease. Primary and secondary prevention strategies running simultaneously will probably have the biggest overall impact.

The techniques described in this book will aid professionals offering individualised counselling for diet and exercise regardless of whether it is part of a primary or secondary approach to prevention. Those in a fitness setting will be more likely to be doing primary prevention work, whereas in healthcare, secondary prevention is more common as professionals tend to be supporting people at risk of, or in the early stages of, chronic disease. Tertiary prevention, which means reducing the morbidity and disability of those with an existing disease, is also likely in the health care setting. An example of this is the advice given about lifestyle change as part of a cardiac rehabilitation programme.

Several large community-based studies have used a variety of different routes in combination to influence and change peoples' lifestyles, and have shown that an effect can be achieved (Puska 1983, Lefebure *et al.* 1987, Murray *et al.* 1990). In North Karelia (Finland), Minnesota (USA) and Pawtucket (USA) different health promotion activities were done simultaneously, including: workplace and school-based health education programmes; mass media campaigns; programmes involving food providers such as caterers, restauranteurs and food retailers; interventions using the health care system; and activities in sports and leisure facilities. In all three studies, the role of health and fitness professionals was an important part of the overall programme of activities but the studies were not designed in a way which made it possible to measure the extent of the success which could be attributed to the one-to-one lifestyle advice given by these two groups of professionals alone.

As mentioned in Chapter 1, some research in the UK has focused on the contribution that one-to-one health promotion advice can make (ICRF OXCHECK Study Group 1994, British Family Heart Study Group 1994). Both the OXCHECK and the British Family Heart studies showed that a small but important effect on CHD risk factors could be achieved after only one year. The changes observed represented an overall reduction in risk of cardiovascular disease mortality of 12%. Both studies ran nurse-led health checks which assessed risk of coronary heart disease and intervened accordingly with all subjects. Investigators in these studies have suggested that a greater effect might have been possible if a more targeted approach had been adopted. If, for example, interventions had been carried out only on those who had been found to be at high risk of coronary heart disease, or with those who had expressed that they were ready to contemplate change, it is likely that the extent of change and the resulting benefit to risk factor status would have been even greater.

Eating

It is clear that dietary advice can have a positive effect on health, but what is less clear is what type of advice, given in what way, is most likely to help. There is growing evidence about the nature of effective nutrition interventions (Glanz 1985, Vickery & Hodges 1986, Longfield 1995), including some from studies involving effective dietary interventions by health professionals or trained lay workers in the primary care setting (Stunkard & Brownell 1986, Ammerman *et al.* 1992, Kyle 1992). A simple overview of dietary counselling is described in Hunt (1995a). A recent report based on a literature review (Longfield 1995) summarises the elements of dietary interventions which have a beneficial effect. They are shown in Figure 3.1 and are described in detail below.

Interesting research by Ormish (1990) shows that with intensive interventions involving a week long residential course, supplemented by two 4-hour group support sessions over a year, an extremely strict diet (vegan, 10% energy from fat) can be achieved, resulting in impressive reductions in blood cholesterol, body weight and other risk factors. But how intensive an intervention needs to be to achieve the less restrictive and acceptable 'healthy diet' which is being advocated is a legitimate question in

Content	Less than 30% energy from total fat and an unspecified or variable energy reduction if weight loss is necessary. Nutrient-based but using foods.
Method of offering:	Relevant printed information *plus* professional. Frequent (with follow-ups) better than one-off. Longer sessions better if possible. Interactive can be better than passive educational style. Must be individualised for client's needs and abilities. Facilitates behaviour change through skills and resources. Use of reinforcement and feedback helps. Include a contract for change.
Source of advice and skills level of adviser:	Appropriately trained health professional. Concern about inadequate knowledge and skill levels of health professionals documented widely. Volunteer (peer) support can be effective.
Recipient of advice:	Higher risk more motivated and successful. Higher educational level more effective. Some prefer groups, some one-to-one.

Figure 3.1 Elements of dietary interventions which have a beneficial effect.

terms of resource allocation. Studies have shown that individual advice given by a dietitian using a tailored diet sheet can be effective (Heller 1989, Cousins 1992) and that additional patient self-help material to use at home can be helpful (Beresford 1992). The duration and frequency of advice-giving sessions, not surprisingly, also has an effect. A series of six or seven follow-up sessions has been shown to be more effective than a single, one-off consultation or group session (Gemson 1990, Iso1991, McGowan 1994).

Interactive educational approaches, particularly those which are computer-delivered, have been shown to have a greater impact on knowledge and self-reported dietary change than passive educational approaches such as lectures or instruction by a video (Kupta *et al.* 1992, Kumar 1993). Finally, Neale (1991) has also demonstrated the effectiveness of encouraging those receiving dietary advice to enter into a 'contract' in which they agree voluntarily to comply with their dietary 'obligations'. 'Contractors' in this study achieved greater beneficial health changes than non-contractors and those who fully met their 'contract terms' experienced the greatest health benefit of all groups.

The practitioner style and skill level has also been shown to have an effect on results of dietary interventions. It has been shown that practice nurses can be trained to offer accurate, good quality dietary advice (Kyle 1993), but concerns remain that members of the primary health care team may lack the necessary skills, knowledge and confidence to offer effective dietary advice (Francis 1989, Cade & O'Connell 1992, Murray 1993). An American study involved dietitians in training to enhance their skills at giving dietary advice (Roach *et al.* 1992). The effects of the training were recorded by videotaping their dietary advice sessions with patients after one week, one month and three months. Some improvements were achieved and the trained groups scored highly on interpersonal skills. There were, however, still areas where improvement was required, including evaluating whether or not the patient had understood what was said, probing about any difficulties patients may have had in following advice and offering strategies to help patients cope with difficulties.

A review of attempts at educational interventions for cardiac patients has concluded that a multi-faceted approach has the best overall effect (Mullen 1992). An optimum educational approach would involve:

- using reinforcement;
- giving feedback;
- offering the opportunity for individualisation;
- facilitating behaviour change through use of skills and resources; and
- the education being relevant to the patient's needs and abilities.

Ramsay and colleagues (Ramsay *et al.* 1991), in a review of the efficacy of studies designed to change dietary behaviour, noted that 'the actual changes in risk factors following the prescription of a particular diet was smaller than expected'. The authors suggest that the diet followed by the subjects was not in line with the regime which had been 'prescribed'. This approach can be questioned. It is possible that it was the quality of the practitioner's advice which was at fault rather than the client's so-called compliance. This review and other reports (Health Education Authority 1993, Department of Health 1994a,1994b) have suggested that further research should be undertaken to identify effective intervention strategies for dietary change. What is clear, is that simple information-giving using a standard leaflet is not sufficient (Thomas 1994).

Exercise

To date there are no published trials of primary care physical activity interventions. In a review of all randomised controlled trials of physical activity promotion (not just those in primary care) only ten trials worldwide were identified. Nine were from the USA, one was from Switzerland and there were none from the UK (Hillsdon *et al.* 1995). A recent review of physical activity interventions in primary care published by the Health Education Authority found a variety of models in operation (Biddle & Fox 1994). The majority involved the referral of patients by a general practitioner (or other health professional) to a leisure centre at a reduced rate for a fixed period of time, typically 10 weeks. Such schemes were usually managed by the leisure centre, who offered low-cost exercise to patients attending with a prescription from their general practitioner (GP). Other schemes identified included: GPs counselling patients on physical activity; a twice weekly outpatients' exercise clinic managed and run within the practice; and a health centre-community project involving practice nurses counselling patients on physical activity and making them aware of all the exercise opportunities within the local community.

The effectiveness of any of these schemes is difficult to assess because they have not been evaluated. Participants in such schemes tend to report favourable responses, such as 'feeling better', 'enjoyment' and 'meeting new friends'. Anecdotal data collected suggest good compliance with the programmes, with many people continuing at the leisure centre on completion of the prescription period. One major drawback of the so-called 'exercise prescription' schemes is the low number of participants upon which the scheme impacts. The HEA report found that less than 1% of a general practitioner's patient list will be involved in such schemes.

The lack of good quality trials in the UK leaves us to draw what we can from work in the USA. In the review by Hillsdon *et al.* (1995), evidence was found to suggest that it was possible to increase physical activity levels in sedentary men and women. There were a number of common factors in the studies that reported significant, positive changes. It appears that physical activities which are home based (e.g. walking, cycling, stair climbing), convenient and enjoyable are more likely to be sustained than structured, supervised, facility-dependent activities. No evidence was found for the effectiveness of programmes that required people to attend a facility (e.g. gym or leisure centre) or structured classes. The average frequency of exercise at follow-up was approximately 2–3 times per week.

In a review of 20 studies of the effect of physical activity and exercise interventions, evidence was found to support the promotion of physical activity. The authors concluded that exercise frequency can be increased but not exercise intensity and that small changes in fitness can be achieved (Dishman & Sallis 1994).

So far, in the field of physical activity, we have been able to show that increasing physical activity levels in people who are sedentary can be achieved and that doing so will produce significant benefits to their health. What we have not done is describe the factors which seem to be associated with achieving change.

Over the last few years a number of reviews of physical activity interventions have been carried out in an attempt to learn more about the adoption and maintenance of physical activity programmes. Perhaps the most comprehensive is that of Dishman and Sallis (1994). A summary of their findings is in Table 3.1.

Table 3.1 Factors associated with the adoption and maintenance of physical activity (adapted from Dishman & Sallis 1994).

Factors positively associated with physical activity	Factors negatively associated with physical activity
Intention to exercise	Lack of time
Expect health and other benefits	Perceived effort
Self-motivation	
Self-efficacy	
Past participation	
Social support	
Enjoyment	
Access to facilities	

It can be seen from the table that exercise programmes should be enjoyable, provide some valued benefit, not be too time consuming and should be easily accessible. Those most likely to engage in such programmes perceive themselves to be fit and well, have previously taken part in some physical activity, are self-motivated and confident about physical activity and have support from family and friends. The authors also found that the inclusion of a behaviour modification component (e.g. relapse prevention) within physical activity programmes was associated with an increase in frequency of physical activity over time.

The review by Hillsdon *et al.* (1995), which was limited to randomised controlled trials in apparently healthy adults, came to similar conclusions as Dishman & Sallis (1994). They found that the intervention most likely to achieve changes in physical activity is: home-based, moderate intensity exercise that can be performed alone or with others, is enjoyable and convenient, and can be completed in three sessions per week. The type of exercise most likely to achieve these criteria is walking. There is some evidence that instruction about self-monitoring and relapse prevention (a behavioural technique aimed at improving maintenance) may improve early adherence. The scenario described could be achieved by an initial brief instructional session followed by short but frequent support, which could easily be provided via the telephone. This approach is low cost and easy to administer compared to facility-based group exercise interventions where the various barriers and costs associated with attendance may lead to high drop-out rates.

This review also highlighted the importance of support, particularly on-going support, in promoting long-term changes in exercise behaviour. The manner in which the health or fitness professional interacts with a client may be the single most important factor for success in one-to-one settings. Researchers in addictive behaviours have suggested that the way in which a therapist interacts with a client may be the best predictor of treatment outcome regardless of any client characteristics, or the particular theoretical orientation of the therapist. A study of changes in drinking behaviour found that half of the variance (difference between groups) in drinking outcomes at 12 months could be predicted from therapist empathy. A recent review of variations in therapist effectiveness with substance use disorders concluded that variations in therapist effectiveness appear to be independent of patient factors and is more to do with the qualities and skills of the practitioner (Najavits & Weiss 1994). They found that the main therapist characteristic associated with high effectiveness is the possession of strong interpersonal skills.

These two reviews provide good evidence as to the type of interventions for physical activity that might be effective for lifestyle change in a primary care setting. An initial brief face-to-face consultation, followed by regular support, focusing on home-based physical activity delivered by staff trained in good negotiating skills and using basic techniques from the behavioural sciences, may be as effective as any more elaborate approach for one-to-one interventions. This will be discussed more fully in Part Three.

External factors influencing change

Clearly changing eating and exercise habits is affected not only by internal factors but also by external factors, some of which are beyond an individual's control. Many of these factors are perceived as barriers to change, while others can be helpful in triggering thinking about change, making it or sustaining it. Cost, access, weather, time of year, food labelling, quality of local recreation services and government policy for example, can all make change more difficult. As this book is primarily about developing strategies to improve the effectiveness of one-to-one counselling, a detailed discussion into these issues will not be undertaken here. However, the management of such difficulties, when presented by clients as barriers, will be discussed in Part Three.

Summary

So far we have shown that evidence exists to support efforts aimed at modifying the population's eating and exercise habits and that achieving such changes would result in significant health and functional benefits. We have also shown that there is now a clear message for both eating and physical activity as to the nature and extent of the required changes. For eating, the *Health of the Nation* and COMA documents provide clear targets which include reducing total and saturated fat intakes and the prevalence of obesity. For physical activity we are guided by the public health policy statement issued from the American College of Sports Medicine and the Centers for Disease Control in the USA, which states that 'every US adult should accumulate 30 minutes or more of moderate intensity physical activity on most, preferably all days of the week'.

The amount of change required to achieve health and functional benefits (such as 'ability to climb stairs unassisted') is clear, but what remains less clear is how to achieve these changes. In the area of dietary change it appears that a practical, food-based approach which takes account of an individual's circumstances, allows scope for flexibility, is tasty, filling, enjoyable and possible for the whole household to take on, is most likely to be sustained. The intervention most likely to achieve changes in physical activity is: home-based, moderate intensity exercise that can be performed alone *or* with others, is enjoyable and convenient, and can be completed in three sessions per week. The mode of exercise most likely to achieve these criteria is walking.

For both food and exercise, the inclusion of some behaviour modification techniques seems to improve the early adherence with on-going support and reinforcement appearing to improve longer term adherence. These changes may be best achieved by an initial brief instructional session followed by short but frequent support, possibly by telephone.

Some indication of the role of the health professional in achieving changes in eating and exercise behaviour has been given but what appears to be lacking at this point is a framework for practitioners to work within which will guide them through the difficult change process and help bring all the successful components of the research into one model. Fortunately, some work in this area has already been carried out. A model of behaviour change which will provide the framework for the rest of this book is described in the next chapter.

Chapter 4
A Model for Change

Unfortunately, the most likely outcome of any attempt to change health behaviour is relapse. That is, a failure to adhere to the intended new behaviour pattern and a move back in part, or more fully, towards the old behaviour. Also, despite a proliferation of formal programmes, most people who make changes in one or more health behaviours do so on their own. In an attempt to learn more about how people change, two researchers from the field of addictive behaviours studied both self-changers and those who attended therapy to attempt stopping smoking (Prochaska & DiClemente 1983). As a result of their studies Prochaska and DiClemente have proposed a model called the transtheoretical model. One of the major themes of this model is that behaviour change involves movement through a series of stages before change is achieved. These stages appear to exist for both self-changers and those attending a treatment programme. In the early development of the model, the following four stages were described.

Precontemplation

This is the stage in which people are not seriously considering the possibility of change. This may be because they are unaware of the existence of a problem or they resist confronting the problem. People in precontemplation are unlikely to attend a formal group or one-to-one counselling session and if they do, it is probably reluctantly due to the persuasion of some other.

Contemplation

This is the stage where people become aware or acknowledge the existence of a problem. They are seriously considering the possibility of change. This stage is characterised by people's ambivalence about change. Although they may see many benefits from changing they are often distressed about what they may have to give up to achieve change. This tussle with the advantages and disadvantages of change can mean that people stay in this stage for long periods of time. They are very open to information about the problem and how it may be changed, and may spend long periods of time trying to fully understand all aspects of it. Prochaska (1994) has found that self-changers for smoking can contemplate the possibility of quitting for 12–24 months before taking action. In practice it is common to hear comments such as 'I know I ought to stop but I haven't quite got round to it yet' or 'I'll start my diet next week'. Next week never comes.

Action

This is the stage when people actually start making some changes in their behaviour. The action stage tends to be the shortest of the stages, lasting up to six months. Other people are often very aware of the person's attempts at change as they seek reassurance and reinforcement for their efforts. It is common for people in the very early part of action to be confident in their ability to sustain change. However, moving into the action stage does not guarantee success.

Maintenance

This is the stage where people attempt to continue with or sustain the progress that they achieved during action. An important component of the maintenance stage is the avoidance of 'slips' or relapse to a less desirable behaviour. People in maintenance, particularly those who have made many change attempts, are often anxious about relapsing. Although they may be doing well at any given time, they constantly struggle with thoughts of relapsing and the temptation to relapse.

Preparation

Following more detailed work on the model, Prochaska (1994) added a fifth stage, the *preparation* stage. This stage lies between contemplation and action. People in the preparation stage have decided to make a commitment to change. Most people in this stage will make an attempt at change in the very near future (within three months). People in this stage, although committed to change, are still ambivalent about it and are still engaging in decision making processes. This means that change is not inevitable and care is required not to hurry these people into action.

Other aspects of the model

Two possible outcomes can result from maintenance. The first is *relapse*. Although this is sometimes described as a stage, it is really a process by which people move back to one of the other four stages. Most relapsers move back to contemplation. In other words, an unsuccessful attempt at change will often result in serious intentions to make another attempt in the near future. Relapse can have a detrimental psychological effect on people which may influence further attempts at change. Feelings of failure can lead to low self-esteem, low confidence and a sense of hopelessness.

The second outcome that may follow on from maintenance, usually perceived as the more successful, is *termination*. Termination occurs when the person is free from the temptation to return to old behaviours and is not continually struggling to ward off relapse. The new behaviour is now more habitual than the old. An example of someone who has 'terminated' the change process is an ex-smoker who no longer refers to herself as an ex-smoker giving up, but a non-smoker. Termination is obviously difficult to achieve and may never be achieved by some people. Even successful behaviour changers can stay in maintenance for ever, always seeing themselves as still changing, having never quite broken free of temptation and never feeling 100% confident about avoiding relapse.

Movement through the different stages towards change is, in general, not linear. Some people may move from 'precontemplation' to 'contemplation' to 'preparation' to 'action' to 'maintenance' to 'termination' without many complications, but most take a more complicated route. Some precontemplators will never move into the change cycle, they remain smokers until they die, or they never take any exercise or attempt to improve their diet. Some people get stuck in 'contemplation' and are always thinking about changing but never quite get round to it. Others constantly take 'action' but never progress to 'maintenance', such as chronic dieters. They are always making a new attempt at losing weight without ever maintaining any losses achieved. For this reason the stages of change are often shown as a circular model rather than a linear one (See Figure 4.1).

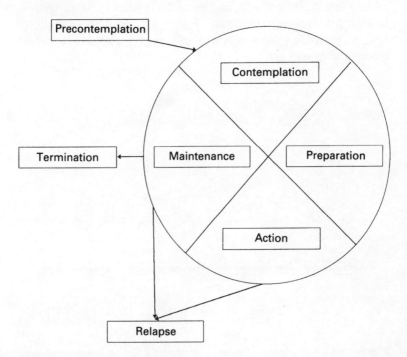

Figure 4.1 Stages of change.

Exit to relapse can occur from any of the stages. A person may enter the cycle at 'contemplation'. After spending time weighing up pros and cons of change, they may decide they don't want to change and exit the cycle. Another possibility is to enter the change cycle at 'contemplation', weigh up the pros and cons of change and move to 'preparation', making a commitment to change. After considering the options for change the person may believe that he cannot successfully carry out any of the options and subsequently give up, leaving the cycle. People in 'action' may decide that the immediate consequences of change are so undesirable that the best choice is to go back to their old ways. Finally, people who have progressed to 'maintenance' may be frustrated at the continued difficulty of sustaining change, expecting things to become easier with time. When things don't become any easier, they decide that the effort to continue doesn't meet with just rewards.

Once they have relapsed people can re-enter the change cycle at any of the stages, depending on where they left it. Or they may not wish to risk further relapse and leave the change cycle altogether, returning to 'precontemplation'. Figure 4.2 gives an example of somebody making three attempts at changing a behaviour before meeting with success.

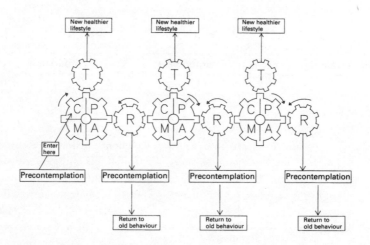

Figure 4.2 Multiple change attempts. C = contemplation; P = preparation; A = action; M = maintenance; T = termination; R = relapse.

The following case study illustrates a movement through several of the stages of change: precontemplation, contemplation, pre-contemplation; contemplation, preparation, action, contemplation; preparation, action, maintenance and termination.

Case study

Mary had got out some of her clothes from last summer in antici-pation of her forthcoming holiday. She decided to try some on to see which things she might like to take with her. To her surprise none of the clothes she tried on fitted, which prompted her to think about the possibility of losing some weight before her holiday. At her first entry to the change cycle she decided that she hadn't really put on much weight, and anyway it was quite nice to have an excuse to buy some new clothes. The prospect of giving up some of her favourite foods and taking some exercise wasn't worth the effort just for a week's holiday. Mary therefore left the change cycle and returned to 'precontemplation'. She went on the holiday, which was with some friends she hadn't seen for a couple of years.

On the first day at the beach, Mary's friends hinted at how much weight she'd put on since they last saw her. Mary got really upset with herself about this which led her to think again about the possibility of losing some weight. This time Mary decided that the benefits of change outweighed the costs and made a commitment to change. She considered her options and decided to start action by cutting out the sweets in her diet and reducing her fat intake. Mary soon became frustrated at not being able to eat the chocolates that she particularly enjoyed and slipped back to her old ways. She still thought losing weight was important and returned to 'contemplation'.

After another few months in contemplation Mary noticed she'd gained a bit more weight and decided to have another attempt at losing some. This time she decided not to cut out chocolate altogether, but to limit herself to two bars a week. She would also cut back on her fat intake, which wasn't too difficult before, and walk to the train station in the morning instead of getting her husband to give her a lift. This would add about 20 minutes of exercise to each week day. Mary continued with this for 6 months and lost a stone in weight. She was very pleased and moved into maintenance, keen to maintain her losses. This she did, finding that she didn't even feel tempted towards chocolate twice a week and the walk to the station had become the norm. She terminated the change cycle with new eating and exercise habits.

This example hopefully helps to demonstrate the dynamic nature of the change process and shows that people can move in and out of the process with a number of different behaviours over short and longer time scales. From their research with smokers Prochaska and DiClemente found that smokers went round the cycle an average of four times before quitting for good. This confirms that relapse is a perfectly normal part of the change process, with each attempt at change increasing the likelihood that the next one will be successful. It does not mean that relapse is inevitable but hopefully helps people to keep it in perspective and use it as a learning opportunity. More details about each of the stages will appear in subsequent chapters.

Processes of change

The stages of change can be seen as markers for different phases of the change process and are an index of when people change. To be better placed to help people in their efforts at change, health and fitness professionals need to know how people change. In the transtheoretical model, the overt and covert techniques and strategies used by people to modify their problem behaviours are known as the processes of change and are an index of how people change. Again, from their work with self-changers for smoking, Prochaska and DiClemente have identified 10 common processes that are consistently used by people giving up smoking on their own or by therapists working with them. The 10 processes are:

1 *Dramatic relief* – experiencing and expressing feelings about one's problems.
2 *Consciousness raising* – increasing information about oneself and the problem.
3 *Self re-evaluation* – assessing how one feels and thinks about oneself with respect to a problem.
4 *Environmental re-evaluation* – considering and evaluating how one's problems affect the physical and social environment.
5 *Self-liberation* – making a commitment to change and believing in ability to change.
6 *Social liberation* – being aware of options and availability of alternative problem-free behaviour in society.
7 *Counter conditioning* – substituting alternatives for the problem behaviour.
8 *Stimulus control* – avoiding stimuli that elicit the problem behaviour.
9 *Reinforcement management* – rewarding oneself or being rewarded by others for making changes.
10 *Helping relationship* – being open and trusting about problems with someone who cares and receiving support from important others.

The practical application of these processes will be described in detail in later chapters.

One of the most important findings from Prochaska and DiClemente's (1984) research, which has important implications for working with people attempting change, is that particular processes of change are emphasised at different stages. Linking the stage of change with the appropriate processes can help us to intervene more effectively with clients. Table 4.1 shows which processes are emphasised at which stages. All 10 processes of change are used least by precontemplators, whereas the experiential (cognitive or thinking) processes (dramatic relief, consciousness raising, environmental re-evaluation, self re-evaluation, self and social liberation) peak during contemplation and preparation, and the behavioural processes (reinforcement management, helping relationships, counter conditioning and stimulus control) peak during the action and maintenance stages. The processes are not applied rigidly to the stages as there is some overlap between them.

Table 4.1 Stages and processes of change

Stage	Processes emphasised
Precontemplation	Processes emphasised least
Contemplation	Dramatic relief Consciousness raising Environmental re-evaluation Self re-evaluation
Preparation	Self-liberation, social liberation
Action	Reinforcement management Helping relationships Counter-conditioning
Maintenance	Stimulus control

The model proposes that matching the right processes to the right stage (often called stage-matching) will increase the likelihood that a person will successfully move through the stages of change. Using the wrong processes and not linking them to the appropriate stage is more likely to lead to premature relapse.

So far, each of the stages of change has been described as a discrete, concrete phase. However, there is in fact, much overlap between them. In practice, it may be useful to view the stages as indicators of 'readiness' to change, on a continuum going from 'not ready at all' (precontemplation), to 'ready' (preparation), through to 'changing' (action). To help us understand the role of the practitioner at each of the stages we will continue to treat the stages separately.

The original development work for the model was based on findings from studies of smokers, but the model has now been applied to 12 different health behaviours, including exercise, high fat diets and weight control (Prochaska *et al.* 1994). Work in each of these 12 health behaviours has provided some evidence to support the generalisation of the model to a range of health behaviours. Interestingly, other theories about behaviour change, such as self-efficacy, relapse prevention and decisional balance, can be integrated into the stage model. This model is truly transtheoretical. That is, it includes elements from and can apply to a wide range of different models of behaviour change and counselling. Although there is substantial research evidence supporting the transtheoretical framework, there is, however, a lack of more powerful clinical trials. Nevertheless, we feel the existing research and the helpfulness of the framework in understanding how people change, justifies its use in practice. The rest of this book will focus on the practical application of the transtheoretical model to the modification of eating and exercise behaviours in one-to-one consultations.

Part Two
A Framework

Chapter 5
Practitioner Qualities

The stages of change model, which is fully explained in Chapter 4 of Part 1, has been chosen as the basis for the brief interventions for lifestyle change described in this book. We have found it to be a most helpful framework. The model is transtheoretical, that is, it draws from and can be applied to a range of different theoretical models and counselling styles. It selects its different component parts from various schools of counselling psychology.

In the approach we recommend the practitioner does not assume an authoritarian role which implies 'I am the expert and I'll tell you how to change your diet or exercise habits'. Responsibility for change is with the client and clients are free to choose to take your advice or not. The strategies used are more persuasive than coercive and more supportive than argumentative. The initial goal is to increase the client's internal motivation, rather than simply trying to impose it from the outside. The next steps involve building confidence for change and negotiating a plan. If done properly this approach means that the client presents the arguments for change and the specific types of changes which seem possible, rather than the practitioner. The interview proceeds with a strong sense of purpose, clear strategies and skills for pursuing that purpose, and a sense of timing to intervene in particular ways at incisive moments.

It follows that in the role taken on in helping people change eating or exercise behaviour, the health or fitness professional could aptly be described as a 'counsellor' or 'therapist'. We prefer to think of them, however, simply as a 'professional helper', as their role is exactly that. For ease the generic, and perhaps less stigmatised, term 'practitioner' will be used throughout this book.

The components of a helping relationship have been much debated over the years and studies have been done in an attempt to identify the best counselling methods or the most effective style.

What exactly is it that makes a helping relationship work? How is a client in need of help, best helped? What are the key things which result in the best outcomes? How much of the success is dependent on the practitioner's style, personal skills and experience? Does it really depend on the clients' characteristics, their starting points or their goals? Or is it primarily dependent on the particular counselling method employed or type of treatment being adopted?

These are not easy questions to answer because controlled and unbiased studies are very difficult to conduct in this field. Reviews of the evidence to date, however, show that perhaps the single most important factor for an effective helping relationship is the practitioner's possession of strong interpersonal skills (Najavits & Weiss 1994). This seems to be the case regardless of their theoretical orientation, the methods they use, the level of training they have received or their experience. The reviews endorse the need for essential practitioner characteristics which were first articulated by Carl Rogers in the late 1950s. The core qualities which appear to be linked to helping are:

1   *Unconditional acceptance* – accepting clients with no strings attached, no matter what their condition, thoughts, behaviours or feelings and not judging them by some set of rules or standards. Respecting them, warts and all. Putting all biases and prejudices to one side. Acceptance should not be confused with approval or liking. This can mean that you do not necessarily like certain aspects of clients or approve of what they do.

2   *Genuineness or congruence* – being freely and deeply ourselves, and able to relate to people in a sincere and non-defensive manner. Genuineness is being real.

3   *Being empathic* – being able to appreciate a client's personal meanings and understanding the world through the client's eyes. This can be done by careful listening and accurate reflection of what you heard, and accompanying the client as he or she progresses through the process of changing.

The focus for the practitioner in the consultation is on entering the client's frame of reference and understanding and tracking the personal preferences, wishes, wants, concerns and difficulties. In essence an effective practitioner accepts all clients unconditionally and believes that they are capable of taking responsibility for their own decisions and actions. If the practitioner qualities described above are in place, change is more likely than if they are not.

The therapeutic alliance

The quality of the relationship between practitioner and client is at the heart of the helping role. This is sometimes referred to as 'the therapeutic alliance'. In his classic text *The Skilled Helper* Egan (1994) proclaims the term 'therapeutic alliance' because it so aptly implies hard work on the part of both practitioner and client as well as denoting a pragmatic partnership, which is related to results.

Only if the practitioner qualities described above are in place, that is, a therapeutic alliance has been formed, will a client feel listened to, understood and trusted. Without them it is doubtful that progress and change for the client will ever occur. It is worth taking the time and trouble to really get to grips with the three qualities which are the essence of the therapeutic alliance, unconditional acceptance, genuineness and empathy. What do they *really* mean? What's behind them? Why are they *so* important? What *skills* does the practitioner need to be able to demonstrate them?

What they show is that you are truly there for people, to help them work through their particular problems. They mean that clients really sense that you are with them and genuinely want to understand them so that you can help. You show that you have understood by listening very carefully, by reflecting back what you think you heard, and checking out with them that your understanding was accurate; you are empathic. So, empathy and reflective listening should be used throughout the whole helping process to show that you accept and understand a client's perspective. Note that this does not mean you have to agree with it.

Active and reflective listening is quite a skill and if done well is extremely effective. To give a client the sense that you really are listening and that you really do want to try to understand their perspective, can be quite novel for them. They may feel that no one has ever genuinely listened or wanted to truly understand their viewpoint before. Paradoxically, this kind of acceptance and respect for people *as they are*, supports their self-esteem and seems to free them to consider change. Conversely, consistent non-acceptance which gives the client a message of, 'you're not OK, you have a problem and you really must change' can have the opposite effect and lead to resistance. Empathic helpers show clients that their perspective is understandable and valid and that ambivalence is accepted as a normal part of anyone's thinking about change. There are always good reasons not to change and good reasons to change and a degree of reluctance to change is absolutely normal.

Although some of the necessary skills for a professional helper might come naturally to you or appear to be plain common sense, others will be more difficult. It's worth taking the time to develop them by attending relevant training courses or practising them with colleagues. You may also consider tape recording some of your sessions so that you can assess how you're doing. Transcribing the tapes, not just listening to them, will really help you to assess the type of questions you asked, what line you were taking throughout the consultation, and how clients responded. Always ask clients if they mind of course, and explain that the recording is simply for your own benefit, to check your own methods of working, and that everything on the tape will be confidential.

A point which warrants mention here is our decision to exclude warmth from this set of practitioner qualities. The debate about this is helpful in demonstrating our conclusion that it need not be a core quality for practitioners helping people change diet and exercise habits. The case *for* including warmth is that it would seem to be essential for building rapport and is an inextricable part of all of the other three qualities: unconditional acceptance, genuineness and empathy. Warmth is a physical expression of understanding and caring which are vital qualities of a professional helper.

An argument *against* warmth is the danger that clients assume it indicates approval, which in turn becomes a false 'hook' in the helping relationship, such that clients never find the means of succeeding without the support of their kind practitioner. This is a dangerous scenario and commonly results in relapse when the sessions end. Warmth can also be misread in other ways. Some clients can find it rather insincere and assume that it isn't genuine as it is switched on for each and every client. Others may feel it creates a passive and non-directive climate and they become frustrated by a warm practitioner who smiles and nods a lot and frequently claims to 'hear what they are saying' but never quite seems to get on with the real business, structure the session or move things forward.

In our debates it became clear that the reason warmth may have seemed important is because of what it represents – a genuine desire to understand and accept the client. There we have our answer. These are the very core qualities we already have: genuineness, understanding (empathy) and acceptance. It is quite possible that you could actually be fairly cold, clipped, efficient and business-like, but providing you showed a genuine desire to understand and accept the client, you would probably still have an effective helping role.

The need for accurate empathy cannot be over-stressed so there is no apology for labouring the point. There is still some confusion among helpers about exactly what empathy is but it has been suggested that accurate empathy accounts for 67% of the total effectiveness of a helping relationship (Miller 1983). This makes it an incredibly powerful practitioner quality and tool. It can be used as part of the helping relationship itself, or as part of the process of helping. In the transtheoretical model, the therapeutic alliance, which is largely based on empathy, is considered to be both a precondition for change as well as a process for change. That is, it has to be in place *before* change can take place and it also is used *throughout* the change process. Egan suggests that although empathy is not the miracle pill, its uses are so varied that it can be directly therapeutic itself. He suggests the following uses of empathy:

- to build the relationship;
- to stimulate self-exploration;
- to check understandings;
- to provide support;
- to lubricate communication;
- to focus attention;
- to restrain the helper; and
- to pave the way.

How empathic are you? Some examples follow which show helpful and unhelpful practitioner responses, both of which are equally well-intentioned.

Empathy means being non-judgemental

C: | I've just become so lazy I suppose. It's disgusting really. I just plonk myself in front of the TV with a never ending supply of food around me. At the time it seems comforting but looking at the state of me now it's hard to imagine why. It's been going on for two or three years.

P1: | I see. I can understand how you must feel. It's tempting to be a bit of a couch potato but it clearly hasn't been the answer for you has it? It's obviously just making you miserable.

P2: | So sitting watching television and eating does have some comforts for you and yet it sounds as if it's not getting you where you want to be.

Practitioner 2 neither judges nor condones. By accurately reflecting the patient's feelings and probing gently, the client is encouraged to explore further. Practitioner 1 paraphrases in a way which introduces negative judgement, in the words used as well as the tone, which the client may perceive as mildly patronising.

Empathy means being non-defensive

C: | I'm not really convinced that there's anything you can do for me. I can't get going on a diet and I feel so tired and hungry all the time. Why should I waste my time coming here?

P1: | Well that is entirely your choice. I'm not here to force you into anything, you do what you want.

P2: | I can see that you're frustrated with it but I think if you were honest with yourself you would see that you are the one wasting time. Change doesn't come easily you know and it seems to me that you're just trying to put it off.

P3: | So you can see some reasons to consider changing but you don't think that coming here can help you. Is that right?

Practitioner 3 shows an accurate understanding of the client's thoughts without challenging them. Ending with a question is a way of checking that he heard correctly as well as enabling the client to think further about his sense that it's not working. Practitioners 1 and 2 have fallen into a trap of being defensive and not being able to take negative criticism honestly. It is unlikely that either of these two practitioners would ask themselves if they were contributing to the apparent stalemate.

Empathy means listening accurately and reflecting

C: | I've tried everything, every diet you can imagine and nothing has ever worked for me. I don't even know why I'm trying again. But things are so bad. My weight is the cause of all my problems. My husband always hated me being fat, the kids' friends tease them about me, I can't get any decent clothes and I just don't go out any more because I feel so awful about myself. I have to do something about this problem. I really do. So I'm trying to make a fresh start.

P1: | Oh dear, I can see that your weight causes you a lot of upset and anxiety. Let's hope we can do something to get you on the right track.

P2: | OK, so you feel that being overweight is making you unhappy and you really do want to give it a go this time. So let's go, eh?

P3: | On the one hand you can see a number of disadvantages of your current weight and yet on the other hand you're worried about trying to change because so far you haven't been able to find anything that works for you.

Practitioner 3 has listened carefully to the overall essence of what the client said and reflected back a careful summary of what she thought she heard. It is clear that she recognises the client's ambivalence and hasn't tried to ignore the magnitude of the problem nor give any false hope that she will definitely be able to help. Practitioner 1 failed to hear and reflect back the client's sense of really wanting to do something about her weight problem and took sole responsibility for trying to solve it for her. Practitioner 2 failed to hear and reflect back the client's concerns about succeeding with weight loss and is being inappropriately optimistic and enthusiastic about success.

Empathy means being perceptive

| C: | You know I really am petrified. My father and uncle both died of a heart attack in their 50s and now I've found out about my high cholesterol level I can see I'm destined for exactly the same thing. What about my wife and family? I don't want them to know I'm so worried. It's the uncertainty and not really understanding this thing about risk and how much of it is in your genes and how much you can change by eating healthily and getting more exercise. The doctors never really tell you very much do they?

| P1: | Well let me try and put this all in context for you. The relative risk of you having a fatal myocardial infarction is certainly raised by the fact that it's in your family but there's no doubt you can reduce that risk by increasing your physical activity levels and eating a healthy diet.

| P2: | Yes, I understand your concerns. Maybe you should bring your wife in so that we can have an open discussion about it. I'm sure she'll be very supportive.

| P3: | So clearly you're worried about the possibility of having a heart attack and you think that your cholesterol level may increase the likelihood of that happening. Also, you're unsure about telling your family because you don't want them to become worried as well, and you think it might help if you understood a little more about the risks of heart disease and what you can do to help reduce your own risk.

Practitioner 3 has sensed the client's anxiety, and so rather than trying to move him on or come up with well-meaning answers and solutions, has simply reflected back what was heard, giving the client the opportunity to expand if he chooses, and talk more openly about his concerns. Practitioners 1 and 2 were both trying to be helpful and caring but responded inappropriately. One leapt in with information, which albeit accurate and relevant, was ill-timed when the client was not likely to be in a frame of mind to receive it. The second suggested involving his wife – a solution which the client had already expressed concern about.

Empathy means staying on the right track

| C: | Not looking after myself or getting a grip in the way all of our family are. It's one of those things I've always had difficulty with and in a way I blame my upbringing for that. Do you get my drift? |

| P1: | Uh-huh. |

| P2: | Yes I think I know what you mean. Now shall we move on? |

| P3: | You don't find it easy taking care of yourself, and you think that your upbringing hasn't really helped much. |

Practitioner 3 uses a simple reflection to show understanding. This will help the practitioner–client relationship and encourage the client to continue. Practitioner 1 hoped that by encouraging the client to continue the point would eventually become clear but this could result in much time wasting, going down a path which is not really leading anywhere. Practitioner 2 did not show respect or understanding. Pretending to understand, then suggesting a complete change of direction, will not give a message of understanding or trust. The therapeutic alliance is on shaky grounds.

A final point about the therapeutic alliance is the use of non-verbal skills which can enhance your helping role. Egan (1994) uses an acronym SOLER to summarize them.

S Face the client *squarely* – a posture that indicates your involvement.

O Adopt an *open* posture – to communicate openness and availability.

L *Lean* slightly towards the client – to say 'I'm with you' rather than 'I'm disinterested'.

E Maintain *eye* contact – to say 'I want to hear and understand what you're saying'.

R Try to be relatively *relaxed* – to show that you're comfortable and expressive.

Chapter 6
Structuring Sessions

Patients attending an appointment with a health or fitness professional could be in any of the five stages of change; precontemplation, contemplation, preparation, action or maintenance. The first three of the stages are the more likely. The following chapter gives ideas about how to structure sessions, the start, the middle part and the closing part, regardless of the client's stage of change, as well as providing more detail on 'getting started'.

Aims of the first session

The first part of the initial session involves firstly greeting your client, secondly helping him to express his concerns and thirdly discussing his expectations and agreeing practicalities such as length of sessions, fees (if relevant) and the number of sessions required. Next, an active approach to solving the problem – by defining it, agreeing on the goal and mapping out the process you will use to support the client with change – will give an indication that you mean business. In terms of your style, it should get across the idea that you are listening, interested, understanding and non-judgemental towards the client.

Building rapport is the first and perhaps most important task you face. Establishing rapport means creating a comfortable, relaxed, unconstrained and mutually accepting interaction between yourself and your client. Whilst this clearly depends on both you and the client, there are things you can do to help create the right atmosphere. Rapport has three essential ingredients: harmony, compatibility and the quality of the relationship. Rapport best develops in the presence of active listening, accurate and empathic responding, reflection of feelings, and a sincere desire to understand. Building rapport is never simple and it is more easily lost than achieved. It is always under threat from misinterpretation caused by ineffective listening.

Consider and find ways of asking why your client has sought help at this particular time. What is the significance of it? Why now? There are ways of asking this without the client feeling pinned against the wall. For example, you could ask, with genuine interest, 'I'm really interested to know what got you thinking about changing your diet or getting more exercise'. By taking seriously their current predicament and present needs, you are respecting your client's frame of reference and using the time economically.

Exploring the client's past history is also an important part of the initial consultation. Most of them will already have tried to eat more healthily or take more exercise at least once, if not many times before. They may have tried under their own steam or have had help from another source, be it a professional, a friend or partner or group support. There are good reasons for asking explicitly about clients' previous experiences. The most sensitive way of enquiring about things which haven't been successful is to ask about 'previous attempted solutions', rather than failed attempts. Try to avoid an interrogative questioning style. The following is an example of how a conversation might go.

P: | Have you tried to change your diet in the past?

C: | Well yes, I've tried a few times, but just never really kept at it.

P: | Can you tell me something about those experiences, perhaps?

C: | Well, I did start watching what I was eating through both of my pregnancies. The ante-natal sessions were really helpful and we had a talk from the dietitian. I just wasn't prepared to put the babies' health at risk by not looking after myself. So that was quite easy. But that was over 10 years ago. The doctor did have a go at me last summer and I got into eating more salads and fruit and cut down on the chocolate and fried foods. The thing is, I've just slipped back to my old ways again.

P: | So it sounds as though some things have worked. You seem to need a specific reason to motivate you to change. And you do like having someone to support and encourage you. What else do you find helps?

C: | Well, I do particularly remember the dietitian and the midwife. It was as if they really cared and they had so much information and practical tips about what to eat. That was really helpful. It was the first time I really understood what a balanced diet meant, and how I could achieve it! And my husband was very supportive for a while too, he stopped bringing chips in and bought flowers instead of chocolates as a treat. It really did make a difference. Thinking about it, the doctor never really helped that much, she just used to nag and I felt guilty. In fact, I did it with my sister-in-law for a while and that was quite supportive too. We had a regular plan to go swimming one night a week and to aerobics on Thursday mornings after the weekly food shopping trip. We really kept each other going.

P: | Mmm. I see. Thanks. That's really helpful for me to get a picture of what's worked for you in the past. Now, I'd like us to talk a bit about exactly how I see our meetings taking shape and how I can support you in getting to grips with this diet thing. Also I'd like to say a bit about what I think it involves for you... Would that be OK?

C: | Fine.

Socialising the client and clarifying the agenda must also take place in the first phase of your initial meeting. This is the beginning of the therapeutic alliance so it is especially important to be natural, courteous and welcoming. It is helpful, if possible, to have said something about your way of working when the appointment was made or in an introductory letter, so that it can then be built on in the first consultation.

It is fair and honest for both you and the client to be clear from the outset about the agenda for your helping relationship. The client's ideas about how you can help, how often they will be coming and for how long may well not accord with your own. Some people may expect and prefer you to give them lots of information accompanied by a sheet of strict instructions, others may imagine it to be more of a 'let's talk about it and see how you feel' kind of experience. Some people might expect to see you for an hour once a week over six months or more, others may think their session is just a one-off.

The potential for incorrect assumptions to be made is great and to avoid any mismatch between your ideas and your client's these issues should be aired and resolved. Set the ground rules by saying 'I see my role as this' and 'I see your role as this' and asking if the client agrees. Make it clear that you are not there to solve clients' problems for them nor to rush them into action, but that you may be able to provide them with information and advice, as well as support them through their own decisions and actions. Be clear about your expectation that they will be prepared to undertake tasks, or 'homework' between sessions as a part of the change process. Stress that you want to make sure that you get the most out of the session as it is their session not yours. On the issue of time and timing, for example, you could say 'I suggest that we spend the 20 minutes we have allotted just now and then arrange some follow-up appointments. Most people seem to find that at least four to six visits are helpful'.

Assessing stage of readiness to change and current behaviour

The stages of change model has already been discussed in Part 1 and in earlier parts of this chapter. An important part of the initial consultation is to try to identify which stage of change the client is in. Although there are tools available which can help you to identify a person's stage of readiness to change objectively, these are more suitable for research purposes. In practice, eliciting information about stage of readiness can be done simply by asking. For example, 'On a scale of 1 to 10 where 1 is not at all ready and 10 is definitely ready, where would you say you are at in terms of your readiness to change?' (Rollnick *et al.* 1992). The main thing to avoid is going too quickly and pushing clients towards action. Although it is also unhelpful to go too slowly with clients who are ready for action, it is likely to be less detrimental than going too quickly.

A final point to mention here is that in assessing stage of change, it can be useful to assess current eating or exercise behaviour. This can certainly be helpful if you suspect you have a precontemplator who already thinks they eat healthily or get sufficient exercise. Also, knowing what people are currently doing may quickly allow you to dismiss the action and maintenance stages. This would avoid the possibility for example, that you discuss the benefits of regular exercise with someone who is already exercising five times per week. There are tools available for assessing current behaviour. For diet, the 'What Do You Eat?' questionnaire (WDYE, see Appendix A) or the Dietary Instrument for Nutrition Education (DINE) are useful (Roe *et al.* 1994). For physical activity the 7-day recall, a structured interview, is most commonly used although there are many others (Blair *et al* 1985). A simple self-administered form is shown in Appendix B. Note that the value of this assessment questionnaire at this stage is only to establish a need for change, not to get into detail about the nature of the change that comes after you have successfully moved your client into the preparation and action stages.

Timing

In the primary health care setting, appointment times vary but it is unusual for a practice nurse to book clients in for any longer than 20 minutes at a time; 10 minutes is probably more typical. The health visitor may have a little more flexibility and in cases where the practice nurse and health visitor work together it may be possible to set aside slightly longer appointment times of 30 minutes for this type of health promotion consultation. The approaches advocated in this book recognise the time constraints in primary care, however, and encourage 'brief interventions' which can be done in blocks of time as short as 10 minutes.

A real advantage of the primary care setting is its access to patients over time, usually many years, which means that follow-up visits are fairly easy to arrange. This is particularly helpful as changes in eating and exercise habits are long-term changes and repeated, ongoing encouragement and support has been shown to have a positive effect on adherence. The brief interventions model usually involves a few short consultations, with some 'homework' for patients to do in between. Follow-up is a vital part of this process.

In surgeries or health centres where effective team working is encouraged and good record keeping systems are in place, an added effect can be achieved by having the different staff members giving consistent reinforcement and encouragement. The doctor might say 'I notice that you set yourself some exercise targets when you saw the nurse in the summer. How's that going?' When attending for a tetanus vaccination the nurse might comment 'I can see from your records that you were working towards a goal weight of 11 stone last year. What's been happening on that front?'. Genuine and timely interest which doesn't come across as inappropriate probing or nagging, can be highly supportive and motivational. People are usually pleased about your interest in them and impressed that you have the relevant and up-to-date facts to hand. Computerisation in practices has made this much simpler.

Importance of follow-up

One of the main factors for success in people who maintain a healthier lifestyle is knowing that some form of ongoing support and encouragement is to hand. This could be from a significant other (partner, close friend or colleague) or initially from a health or fitness professional. In the early phases the value of your support through regular follow-up should not be underestimated, even if it is just for a brief, 2- or 5-minute consultation.

An experience one of us has had in developing a 32-page self-help booklet for dietary change reinforced this fact (Hunt 1995d). A short diary section was included to enable clients to monitor their own progress. Immediately after the diary, a section entitled 'When the going gets tough' was included. In the evaluation of the draft booklets the clients rated this particular part of the whole booklet, on how to cope when relapse loomed, as one of the most helpful. Health professionals were asked the same question ('Which sections of this booklet do you think would be the most helpful for clients?') and none of them mentioned this 'support' section. It was a clear indication that for clients, having some sort of immediate support to hand, even only through written material, was highly valued. Yet the health professionals had not recognised the client's need for – and the perceived value of – such support. Follow-up is vital and easily arranged in the primary care and fitness setting. The value of the practitioner's supporting role should not be underestimated.

Finishing sessions

The type of helping relationship you have with your client is not open-ended. You need to develop skills in terminating each meeting appropriately, as well as handling the last in your series of sessions with the client. If you are clear at the outset how long each meeting will be, and how many times you expect to see each other, the finishing process is much easier. Rather than letting the subject of termination slide it is better to keep it alive. Some practitioners find that a countdown system works well. 'So we've now got to the end of our second meeting which means that there are four more to go.' Not least you should keep examining progress with termination in mind because a dependency on you may be partial avoidance of the hard work required by the client to achieve personal change. Some clients would probably continue seeing you indefinitely if it were possible. Reminding them of why they first came, of how much they have achieved and by affirming a belief in the time-limited nature of the help you are offering, may help to make ending sessions more positive.

Chapter 7
Getting Started

Two key factors will influence your introduction, your first question in the consultation and your course of subsequent help. These are how the person arrived with you and what they think they are there for. The set of circumstances will be very different depending on whether you are a health professional or a fitness professional. A fitness professional is much more likely to see clients who are clear about their overall aim, which is usually along the lines of 'to get in shape, get fit, look good, improve health by being more active and, possibly, eating more healthily'.

If you are a health professional the introduction to eating and exercise will probably be much less clear cut and the client may not even have lifestyle issues in mind at the time they first see you. This is discussed more fully in the next few pages.

Getting started in the primary care setting

How you get started will depend on whether the appointment has been arranged especially to discuss a particular health behaviour (be it as a result of a referral from another health professional, a previous consultation with you, or the client's own self-referral) or whether you are raising diet and/or exercise opportunistically.

A planned or arranged session

If it is a planned session, in which the client is fully expecting to discuss healthy eating and/or exercise, the first part of the initial session is relatively straightforward. It is still helpful, however, for both you and the client to be clear about the purpose of the session and what expectations, preferences and concerns you each might have about it. Has the client been shocked by the sudden death of a colleague or neighbour, or coerced into coming by a spouse or family member? Have they been referred to you by the doctor? Establishing a clear picture of this gives some insight into people's expectations and motivations and will enable you to find out about any misconceptions they may have.

Some clients may have come to see you because they've been told they should, but are not really convinced themselves. Others may arrive with the idea that there is something dreadfully wrong with them, which may be based on misinformation. An example is someone with a high blood cholesterol level, discovered through a blood test done at the local pharmacy. He may well be terrified and imagine that unless he makes drastic lifestyle changes immediately he is sure to have a heart attack. He believes, literally, that his life is in your hands. If clients have been referred by a doctor or health professional, what information were they given and what were they told to expect from you?

A useful first question then, both to help establish rapport and also to gain insight into how the client sees your role, is simply to ask 'What is your expectation of what I can do to help you?'. You will quickly find out whether or not clients are attending because they want to and also start to build up a picture of how motivated they are.

An opportunistic session

Raising the issue opportunistically, which is more likely to apply in the health care setting, requires a different set of questions and skills. You can never predict what kind of response you will get. By opportunistically, we mean taking the opportunity at a time when the client has come to see you for something else, be it related (e.g. high blood pressure) or unrelated to general lifestyle issues (e.g. an ingrown toe nail or for contraceptive advice). That is, you are using an opportune moment to raise the important issue of health promotion and suggest that there are lifestyles changes they might want to consider if they wish to look after their own health.

Raising the issue without irritating the client is a real art. There is a fine line between being helpful and being perceived as an imposing busybody who enjoys telling people how to live their lives. 'Advise – yes, dictate – no' is an appropriately titled paper which summarises patients' views on health promotion in the consultation (Stott & Pill 1990). The authors describe the boundaries of advice giving and strongly discourage a dictatorial and instructive style. An approach which implies 'I'm telling you this because I'm a health professional so know how important it is for your health – I really think you should do it', will not help. Although done with the best of intentions the most likely result is feelings of guilt.

Professional dominance, finger wagging and victim blaming do not help. 'Gosh, I see your weight has gone up another five pounds since you were last here; you really are going to have to get it under control aren't you?', will achieve nothing and may well be a retrograde step. Most clients know when their weight is increasing and don't feel good about it. It is most unhelpful to have someone reinforcing their problem, without an offer of support or a hint that weight loss may be possible.

Your challenge is to ask the right questions in the right way. 'I don't know what you make of this, but your weight is currently 12 stone 9 lbs. How does that sound to you?' is a much more helpful way of raising the issue. The response to that question will probably give you a general indication of the client's stage of readiness to change. The following are examples of the types of response you might get from people in the different stages of change.

Precontemplator

'Gosh, I had no idea that it was anywhere near that. I suppose that could mean I'm a bit overweight, does it?'

'That can't be right. Anyway it's never really bothered me. My husband likes me like this and I've always been on the big side.'

Contemplator

'I've noticed that my clothes were feeling a bit tight lately. I really ought to think about tackling it, but I've always found dieting so difficult.'

'You've confirmed what I'd feared I suppose. But wouldn't you expect someone of my age to naturally start getting this middle age spread?'

A preparer

'I know, I've been thinking about it quite a lot lately and have recently made plans with my friend to start going to Weight Watchers. I do hope I can stick at it this time.'

'Yes, we've agreed within the family that we're all going to have a serious attempt, *en masse*, at eating more healthily and getting more exercise. I think we'd enjoy it and would certainly feel better for it. Our goal is to be fit and trim for our holiday in four months time. Do you think we'll succeed?'

A client in action

'Yes I know that's too much, and I have already made a start. In fact, that's already an improvement. Four weeks ago I was almost at the 13 stone mark!'

'Well I've recently changed to skimmed milk and low fat spread and definitely eat less fried food and sweet stuff now. I feel much better for it already but am struggling a bit with some of the changes I've tried.'

A client in maintenance

'I know I'm still quite heavy for my height, but it's much better than it was. We all eat healthily as the norm now and apart from the occasional celebration meal I think I have a very low fat diet. So, for the type of food we eat, I think I'm a convert! However, I've noticed that I've been sneaking in a few extra things lately. Perhaps I need to focus more on the amount of things I'm eating and maybe getting a bit more exercise?'

'I'm really pleased with that, I've been working so hard. The trouble is I'm struggling a bit now. It's getting boring and I keep thinking about all the nice things I miss. I don't want to go back to where I was though.'

From this opportunistic raising of the issue, it will usually be necessary to arrange a follow-up appointment, if the client agrees, to discuss the issues of changing eating and/or exercise habits more specifically. Occasionally you may get a hostile response which indicates that your client is firmly in precontemplation (or possibly that you have attempted to move them on too quickly). The most important thing here is to develop rapport with clients to be non-threatening and to encourage them to consult you again if they feel they would like to consider change.

The nature of the consultation will depend ultimately on which stage the client is in as described in the following chapters. Even within the first 10–20 minutes appointment however, you ought to be able to identify which stage the client is in and possibly help them to move from the stage they are currently in, to the next stage. At the very least you should help clients to clarify issues about the stage they are in and to go away and think about it or do something which may help to move them on. The example given is the start of a session with a practice nurse arranged following referral from the doctor who felt this lady should lose some weight before her forthcoming hysterectomy. The dialogue given is after the initial formalities and rapport building. It aims to find out about her expectations of the session, to get a sense of her degree of readiness and motivation to change and her previous dieting history, if possible. As you read, decide which stage of change you think the client is in.

P: So, do you know exactly why you're here today?

C: Well, the doctor said that I needed to see you to talk about losing some weight before my hysterectomy operation.

P: Okay, and how do you think I might be able to help you?

C: I don't know really ... but I do know I don't want to be nagged at ... and I'd be disappointed if you gave me a diet sheet with lists of do's and don'ts. I've done that before and didn't find it very helpful.

P: So you've tried to lose weight before and found some things didn't work for you.

C: Yes.

P: It would probably be useful at this point for me to explain about how I think we will be working together. I already appreciate the fact that you have made the effort to come here today and it is usual to have three or four sessions together. I should also explain that it's not my job to try and change you. I hope that I can help you think about your present weight and consider what, if anything, you want to do about it, but if there is any changing, you will be the one who does it. Nobody can tell you what to do; nobody can make you change. I'll be giving you information and some advice, but what you do with that after you leave here is up to you. I couldn't change you even if I wanted to. The only person who can decide whether to change and how to change is you. In this first session what I'd like to do is take a close look at your situation and try to understand your weight more. What do you think about that. What would you particularly like to do today?

C: It sounds good, because I thought you might just tell me off for what I eat, you know. I'm not sure if there is anything in particular, just to talk about my weight I suppose.

Most clients will feel a sense of relief after hearing about this approach. However, for some you may need to do some more explaining, especially those who thought that you would just give them a diet sheet or eating plan and that would be it. Some follow-on lines might include:

P: You sound as if you were expecting something else.

C: Yeah, all I need is a plan. You know a diet sheet or something, then I'll do it.

P: In my experience, most people who I have provided diet sheets for do okay for a few weeks, but don't seem to get good results in the long run. What do you think?

C: But I'm more motivated this time.

P: Okay, but the fact that you're here would suggest that this approach hasn't been particularly successful for you either. Do you think that there is any advantage in thinking things through a little to try and improve the prospect of better results in the long run?

C: I suppose there is really, but what else is there I can do. I mean I've tried everything.

On occasions like these, clients are almost destined to fail if they don't prepare well before undertaking a major change such as this.

Prochaska and DiClemente (1984) have pointed out the importance of thorough and careful preparation before moving into the action phase.

Once you have made it clear to the client how you will be working you can continue by trying to understand their situation.

P: Perhaps we can start then, by you telling me what you've noticed about your weight. How has it changed over time?

C: Well I was trim when I got married, then with having the three children it rocketed. I suppose I ate for comfort really – they used to drive me mad when they were little! About 5 years ago I did lose a bit, then put it all back on. Last year I had another real go and got right down to 13 stone. But look at me now, almost back to square one. I don't seem to have the will power.

P: So you gained weight with having the children and while they were young. More recently you have successfully lost some weight, twice. But both times it's gone back on.

C: Yes ... but I'm determined not to give up this time.

P: Okay, tell me a bit about how you managed to lose the weight before.

C: I suppose just by being sensible and cutting out nibbles and snacks between meals. The second time I did calorie counting which did make me realise about all the hidden calories in some things. Quite an education that was!

P: So cutting out the extras and counting calories worked for a while.

C: Yes. And I still remember it all. It's just sticking at it that I find impossible.

P: So you have found some things that have worked for you, but you have found some difficulty sticking to them.

C: Too right.

P: So how does your weight now compare with before?

C: Well, to be honest with you I think I weigh more than ever before. I really do want to shift it.

P: OK, well, just thinking about what you eat currently, what is it that you like about that? And on the other hand, in what way are some of your current habits unhelpful for your weight?

This patient is clearly in 'contemplation'. She is thinking about change but has not yet quite decided to do it. From here you would continue with strategies designed for contemplators, which can be found in Chapter 9. You may find that after taking a history you are close to being out of time. At this point you may ask the client to carry on with some of the processes as homework between sessions. In the dialogue above, it might be useful to set the task of completing a written decisional balance as described in Chapter 9.

Finishing the first session well is as important as starting it well. Try to summarise the major points of the session, agree tasks to be done before next time and ask the client what they did and didn't find helpful.

P: We are just about out of time now, so before we finish I'd like to just summarise what we have covered today. Along with the doctor you also have some concerns about your weight. You have had a number of attempts to lose weight before and have found a number of things to be helpful including cutting out between meal snacks. Also, counting calories helped you to see that some foods were higher in calories than you thought. However, up to now you haven't really found a way that's worked well in the long run. Your weight is now heavier than before and you want to consider what you might do about it. Have I covered everything do you think?

C: Yes, I think so. I do want to get this sorted out and get started.

P: What might be helpful between now and next time is for you to write down a list of advantages and disadvantages of reducing your weight and then do the same for staying the same. You could do it on a sheet like this [shows an example of a decisional balance sheet]. This will help you focus on exactly what you have to gain and also help you see what difficulties there may be. We can discuss these when we meet again. Does that sound like something you could do?

C: Yes, I think so, as long as we can meet again soon.

| P: | Before we end, could you tell me what you found helpful and unhelpful about today? |

| C: | Well, I'm glad that you didn't tell me off and that you didn't just tell me what I was doing wrong, that was good. I don't think there was anything unhelpful apart from I would have liked more time. |

| P: | Yes, that's always a problem. Still, it doesn't stop here. If you would like we can meet again in a week or two and carry on. |

You can see how the rapport has been developed at the start of this consultation, with the client engaged and involved rather than the practitioner doing all the talking. Also the practitioner is genuinely interested in trying to understand the client and her attitudes to and experiences of weight loss. The brief dieting history the client gave indicates that she probably has a fairly good knowledge about the health and nutritional value of foods. She has said several times that she really does want to lose weight, but would find it difficult. She is in contemplation because she has recognised that she is going to have to change her diet to lose weight, which she believes is necessary and has indicated her intentions to do so. However, she clearly needs to consider the difficulties involved before she will commit herself to changing.

There is more about how to continue and end such sessions later in the chapter and in Chapter 9.

Getting started in the fitness setting

In a fitness centre or health club setting, it is common to have an initial consultation with people lasting from 30 minutes to 1 hour. Clients attending these sessions are usually in contemplation or preparation. Some clients may be transferring from another club or facility and may already be in action or maintenance. Very few if any clients will be in precontemplation, mainly due to the requirement to pay to attend such facilities.

With this much time available it is very likely that the practitioner can move through contemplation to preparation in one session. Therefore, the aim of the session should be to build motivation for change, strengthen commitment to change, build confidence for change, discuss options for change and negotiate a plan of action. One helpful way of getting started after the formalities of introductions is to set an agenda for the session. This helps to make the best use of the time available for both you and your client. Clients should be given the first opportunity to set agenda items, encouraging them to be involved right from the start.

P: | We have 45 minutes together today during which time there are a range of things we can talk about. So that we both make the most of the session I usually find it helps to set a bit of an agenda. Is it okay if we do that?

C: | Sure.

P: | Okay, what things would you like to make sure we cover today.

C: | I'd like to talk about my fitness.

P: | What else?

C: | The difficulty I've had keeping going with programmes before because of the lack of time.

P: | That's great. There are a few things I'd like to cover, mainly involving asking you questions that will help me help you as much as I can. Just before we start, is there anything you particularly don't want to do during this session?

C: | I can't think of any just now.

P: | Well, I assume from the fact you are here that you think perhaps you need to make a change in your exercise habits?

C: | Yes, I need to get myself fit and get my weight down a bit.

P: | Tell me a bit about your exercise. How has it changed over the past few years?

C: | I used to be really quite fit, when I was at university I used to train 3–4 times a week.

P: | What kind of things did you do?

C: | Mainly I used to row. I really enjoyed it.

P: | What other things did you do?

C: | That was it basically, although it wasn't all in the boat, we did gym work too. Lifting weights and circuit training.

| P: | You worked hard at it. |

| C: | Yeah. |

| P: | How long did you continue with that for? |

| C: | Well I stopped almost as soon as I left university. You know, new job, new house, etc. |

| P: | Perhaps you could tell me about the amount of exercise you do now. |

| C: | Nothing! |

| P: | And what concerned you about doing nothing that made you think that you ought to make a change? |

You can see how we have encouraged the client to become involved in talking about his exercise, both historically and currently early on in the consultation. The idea is to convey to the client a desire to understand the behaviour from their point of view. A history of taking part in exercise will come in useful when it comes to negotiating a plan. The client will have some idea of the things he does or doesn't like and is more likely to be confident about engaging in exercise than somebody for whom the whole experience is new. The final question by the practitioner is starting to explore reasons for change and build motivation. More details of this can be found in Chapter 9, on contemplation.

Once this has been done and the client has made a strong commitment to change, work can start on negotiating a plan. Again, examples of how to do this can be found in Chapter 10, on preparation.

Closing the session should involve a summary and an opportunity for the client to ask any questions, as shown in the primary care setting example given earlier. You should also ask the client what they found helpful and/or unhelpful about the session. This not only helps you structure future sessions but again indicates to the client that you are interested in helping them.

| P: | We've covered quite a lot of points today, I wonder if it might be a good idea to try and summarise what we've done? |

| C: | Sure. |

P: We discussed the fact that you've exercised in the past but have had a break of about five years and that currently you don't do any exercise. You said that the trigger for you to consider changing now was the fact that you went to have a game of football with your mates, which you haven't done for a long time, and you found it very hard going. That concerned you as you felt that you should be able to do that kind of thing without too much bother. You then said that the things you think you will like about exercise are regaining that kind of fitness and hopefully losing a little weight. You didn't want to stay as you were because you believed that this would mean a further deterioration in your fitness, which isn't good for your health, and you would probably continue to gain weight. How am I doing so far?

C: Fine.

P: We then went on to discuss your concerns about your lack of time and agreed that initially two sessions a week of 45 minutes each were realistic to start with. You agreed that even when you're busy at work you would still be committed to the two days, although you may have to limit the session to 30 minutes. Is that everything?

C: Yes, I think so.

P: Have we covered everything you would have hoped to today?

C: Yes, definitely.

P: What did you find helpful today?

C: Well, I was surprised that you didn't tell me what to do. Initially I was a bit disappointed but now I realise that I'm the one who has to do this and I think that I'm more likely to stick at it because I've come up with the plan. I can't use the excuse that it was someone else's idea, that's why I couldn't do it.

P: What else?

C: That was the main thing.

P: What didn't you find helpful about today?

C: Nothing really. As I say, I thought you were going to do all the work not me, but I realise now that wouldn't have been that helpful in the long run.

Before closing the session don't forget to make a follow-up appointment. This will be influenced by how confident both you and your client feel about implementing the plan. It can be useful to ask the client when this should take place. Typically it will be between 2 and 8 weeks. If the person is new to exercise it is better to do it sooner rather than later.

Negotiating for change is an art not a science and we are therefore reluctant to give rigid and inflexible structures for you to work to. It may be helpful to use the following checklist as a reminder of how to proceed in the initial consultation. Do bear in mind, however, that each client's response will be different and it may throw you off course unless you are skilled enough to be completely flexible and responsive. Practice, practice, practice!

Checklist for the initial consultation

Beforehand

1 Do you have the appropriate practitioner qualities?
2 Have you acquired and practised the basic skills required for an effective helping relationship?
3 Are you prepared to be flexible in your style, to best suit the needs of each client?

The process

1 Have you welcomed your client and established rapport?
2 Are you aware of the context in which he is seeing you? Why now? Who has referred him?
3 Is the client aware of your preferred way of working and your expectations of him?
4 Is the client aware of the length of each session, the likely duration of the whole 'treatment' and your fees?
5 Have you heard (briefly) his story? The problem? His concerns? His past history (what has worked well and what has worked less well for him)?
6 Have you established the client's own diet or exercise-related goals?

7   What is his own assessment of his current dietary or exercise behaviour (see **11**)?

8   Is the client aware of the discrepancy between points 6 and 7?

9   Have you identified the client's stage of change?

10   What is your objective assessment of his current dietary or exercise behaviour and how does it compare with his own in point 7?

11   Have you begun to work with the client on solving the problem? Defining it? Agreeing the goal? Mapping out the process you will use to support the client through change?

Part Three
Practice

Chapter 8
Helping the Precontemplator

Characteristics of the precontemplator

Precontemplators are not seriously considering change. They may be unaware of the existence of a problem, such as not taking regular exercise, or even if they are aware may still be resistant to information about change. They may resist being informed about change for a number of reasons. These include the possibility that change may mean giving up something valuable (such as time spent with the family or relaxing in front of the television) or anxiety about not being able to achieve change even if it was attempted. Anxiety about change is often the case with people who have had many attempts at change, such as chronic dieters, who often make comments such as 'I'll never be able to lose weight, I've tried every programme going and I'm still fat'. They feel unable to control their eating or problem behaviour and feel hopeless about the future. Even if they do attempt change, it is likely to be half-hearted.

Some precontemplators are resistant to change because they don't believe change is necessary. The Allied Dunbar National Fitness Survey revealed that as many as 80% of inactive people believe that they are already fit enough and a similar problem is true for eating; when asked if they would consider themselves to be healthy eaters, over two-thirds of people say 'yes'. Messages to improve fitness and diet, or advertising campaigns giving advice to take more exercise and choose healthier food products will not be heard by these people.

One final reason for not considering change can be that admitting to a problem such as overeating may be seen as revealing a weakness which can lead to loss of self-esteem. Most people are reluctant to admit such weaknesses as they believe that they must be in control of their lives.

Attempts to get precontemplators to change will be interpreted as a threat to their freedom to choose how they behave and to their autonomy, and will be met by resistance and hostility. None of us like being told what to do.

In summary, precontemplators believe that the advantages of staying as they are are greater than the disadvantages, and that the cost of change is greater than the potential benefits. They are not very confident about their ability to change and temptations towards their existing behaviour are very high. The processes of change are used least by precontemplators.

Processes emphasised during precontemplation

These are helping relationships; dramatic relief; and environmental re-evaluation.

Therapeutic goal of the precontemplation stage

To help the client become aware of the existence of the problem behaviour and its accompanying risks through education and feedback. To encourage the client to consider the possibility of change.

Working with the precontemplator

The processes emphasised during this stage are aimed at helping clients to realise the existence of a problem behaviour and its impact on themselves and those around them. This can involve a large amount of information exchange. The way in which information is exchanged can result in either resistance or progression through to contemplation. The outcome will be influenced by both the content of the information and by the way it is delivered.

Information should be shared with the client neutrally. This means that it is important not to evaluate the information on behalf of the client. For example: 'I've taken your weight Malcolm and as you can see it is 16 stone and 4 pounds. This is bad news for your blood pressure, we're really going to have to do something about this'. In this dialogue the professional has decided that Malcolm's weight is 'bad', which is using scare tactics to encourage change. Also, the professional has decided on the client's behalf that he should do something about it, which discourages input from the client and is unlikely to increase self-motivation. The client is not engaged in any aspect of the process and has had no freedom of choice to act on the information.

When feeding back such results there should be an emphasis on freedom of choice and on the client's evaluation of the feedback: 'I don't know whether this will concern you Malcolm, but your weight is 16 stone and 4 pounds ... Is that what you expected? ... How do you feel about this? How do you think that might influence your blood pressure?'.

As mentioned previously, any information relating to change at this point will be premature and is likely to lead to defensiveness from the client. Dramatic relief relates to the person's emotional response to the possible consequences of negative events occurring as a result of the problem behaviour. An example at this point may help to illustrate how these processes relate to an actual situation.

P: I don't know how important you think this is, but your current level of physical activity is low compared to the level that may benefit your health.

C: I've never really done much exercise.

P: Would it be okay if we took a few minutes to discuss it a bit more?

C: Sure.

P: Perhaps we could start by you telling me what you know about exercise and your health.

C: Well, you have to do a lot of it before you get any benefit.

P: But if you did do a lot there are some benefits.

C: Yes.

P: What might some of those be?

C: I suppose you'd feel fitter and you might lose a bit of weight.

P: So you know getting fitter and losing weight can be benefits of taking exercise, what else?

C: I'm not sure really.

P: I've got some information about some other benefits, would you be interested in hearing them?

C: | Okay.

P: | People who exercise regularly compared to those who do no exercise have about half the risk of suffering a heart attack, generally have lower blood pressure, lower cholesterol, manage their weight better, are more able to do day-to-day tasks as they get older, and on the whole feel better than people who take no exercise. What do you make of that?

C: | I didn't know it was that important.

You can see that it was possible to raise the issue and educate the client about exercise without appearing to be coercing him towards change. At no time was there a suggestion that the client must change and he was encouraged to take part in the exchange right from the start. Instead of evaluating the benefits of exercise for the client, he was given the opportunity to express how he felt about them. There are two important points here. One is to raise the issue of the behaviour during the session and the second is to raise the client's awareness of how it relates to him or her. This next dialogue will show an example of this being done from start to finish.

P: | If you remember, as part of your routine health check I asked you some questions about how much exercise you do. I don't know what you will make of this, but in terms of your health you are relatively inactive.

C: | I do as much exercise as the next person.

P: | This isn't what you expected.

C: | I know I don't go to a gym or anything but I'm always on the go.

P: | You think that you probably do enough exercise.

C: | Compared to other people I know, yes.

P: | I wonder if I might take a couple of minutes to explain how much exercise is required to benefit your health.

C: | Okay.

P: | The latest evidence suggests that we ought to do at least 30 minutes of moderate exercise, that's exercise that makes us a bit out of breath and warm, on most days of the week and preferably all days. What do you make of that?

C: Perhaps I'm not doing as much as I thought.

P: How much does that concern you?

C: Well, I've never really thought about it that much before.

P: I suppose it's hard for you to see, especially as you thought you were doing enough exercise.

C: Yes, I mean I don't feel unfit.

P: At the moment you can't see any problems associated with not doing that much exercise.

C: No not really.

P: Has there been a time when you were more active than you are now?

C: Oh, yes definitely

P: What has changed?

C: I used to do a lot of sport up until a few years ago, I was very fit, I played football twice a week and went swimming once a week. But then I moved and never got round to finding a new club.

P: What did you like about doing those things.

C: I had quite a few friends and felt a bit more energetic than I do now. I've gained a bit of weight since then as well.

P: How much does your weight gain and lack of energy concern you?

C: Now that I'm thinking about it, I suppose it would be nice to feel that fit again and lose a few pounds.

P: What else did you like about being that fit.

C: Just the social part really.

P: You enjoyed the camaraderie of playing sport.

C: Yes.

| P: | If you were to make a change how would you hope to benefit. |

| C: | Well, I would definitely feel fitter and I'd hope to get my weight down a bit. |

| P: | What else? |

| C: | If I found a good club, then maybe I'd meet some new people. |

| P: | And you'd like that. |

| C: | Yes. |

| P: | I'm conscious that we're running out of time and I wondered if I might just summarise what we've done today. |

| C: | Sure. |

| P: | First of all I told you that your current level of physical activity isn't benefiting your health as much as it might, which you were surprised at. You thought you were quite active, especially compared to some people you know. We then looked at how much exercise is ideal and you realised that it was quite a bit more than you do at the moment. You then told me about how fit you've been in the past and that when you were that fit you had more energy, were a bit leaner and you enjoyed the company of the people you were with. You also said that if you were to become more active now you would hope to feel fit again, lose some weight and hopefully meet some new people. Is that everything, or do you think I've missed anything. |

| C: | No, that's what we said. |

| P: | Where do you think we go from here. |

| C: | I'm not sure. |

| P: | Perhaps we could meet again in a month and during that time I could give you some information to read about some of the other benefits of becoming more active. Do you think you might do that? |

| C: | Yes, okay. |

You can see from this consultation that the client was gradually moved along towards contemplation. By using open-ended questions and accurate reflection the professional was able to help the client see the need to consider change. If we remember that the aim of this session was to move on one stage then it could be regarded as a success. Obviously there are many different ways this consultation could have gone. For example, it might have been necessary to focus more on the consequences of inactivity to provoke an emotional response from the client. Be careful, though, not to appear to be threatening the client if you adopt this approach, for example 'If you don't take more exercise you're likely to end up having a heart attack'. It is better for the helping relationship to have the client consider the consequences of inactivity: 'What do think might happen if you continue as you are?'.

Sometimes, occurrences in the environment can lead to an emotional response in clients. Dramatic relief can be provoked by a relative or close friend having a heart attack. The resulting anxiety may lead the person to seriously consider their own health and the possibility of changing their lifestyle. It is this kind of event in someone's life that is often what moves them out of pre-contemplation. Although practitioners can't create such events, they can help the client make the link between them and their behaviour.

Throughout this stage, the professional should always have in mind that the aim is to move on one stage and should be careful to avoid rushing the client towards action.

Chapter 9
Helping the Contemplator

Characteristics of the contemplator

The contemplator has recognised the existence of a problem behaviour and is seriously considering the possibility of change but has not yet made a commitment to change. Contemplators are open to new information and often actively pursue it in an attempt to understand the problem and how it may be resolved. They wrestle with the positive aspects of changing on the one hand, and on the other, the time, effort, energy and potential losses required to achieve the positive things. They are said to be ambivalent about change and are constantly weighing up both the pros and cons of their existing behaviour and the pros and cons of change. 'I know it would be better if I cut down on my fat intake, but I really like butter and I couldn't possibly go without my afternoon cake. I'd probably feel better if I could change, but it all seems such hard work.'

People can become stuck in contemplation for months and years. They are frequently heard talking about change but are slow to take action. 'I really ought to take some more exercise, but I never seem to have the time', or 'I bought a new exercise video last week but haven't got round to watching it yet'. Many people have bought home exercise equipment and never used it.

Some people become frustrated in contemplation because they are highly motivated towards two highly desirable and yet opposing states. An example would be wanting to be slim and yet wanting to continue to eat all of their favourite foods (which probably includes high fat and sugary foods). Such people talk about the unfairness of the situation and wish there was an easy solution which would allow them to have both states. You may often hear them refer to their friends who seem to be able to eat all they want and still stay slim. They will put off change in the hope that a simple solution will arrive, 'I'll do it tomorrow', in the hope that tomorrow will somehow be easier, but it never is.

In summary, contemplators see the pros and cons of changing and the pros and cons of staying the same as equal and consequently are ambivalent about change.

Processes emphasised during contemplation

Consciousness raising, dramatic relief, environmental re-evaluation, self re-evaluation.

Therapeutic goal of the contemplation stage

To understand the client's ambivalence and tip the balance in favour of change. To build confidence for change and achieve commitment to change.

Working with the contemplator

The contemplator is struggling with the conflict of recognising that there may be significant benefits arising from making changes, yet also recognising that change may also mean giving up something of value. Self re-evaluation, one of the most important processes during this stage, is an emotional and rational appraisal of both the pros and cons of change and the pros and cons of staying the same. Environmental re-evaluation, another process emphasised in this stage, is the appraisal of how the client's current behaviour effects others around them, as well as how a change in behaviour might also affect others. This information is included in the weighing up of pros and cons. This can be particularly important when contemplating changes in eating behaviour. If the person considering change is the primary cook in the family, then changes in his or her own behaviour will have an immediate impact on others, which may be good or bad. This conflict between the pros and cons is the the essence of ambivalence, the co-existence of feelings that are conflicting with each other. An example is the yo-yo dieter. They alternate between the desire to be slim, resisting cues to eat high fat and calorie dense foods, and the desire to continue to eat their favourite foods, resulting in over-indulgence in them.

This wavering between the costs and benefits of change and no change is what characterises this stage and it is the professional's role to try and understand it and not confront it. It may be also be necessary to provide the client with information to help with decision making. This is the process 'consciousness raising', which involves education and feedback about the client's current behaviour. 'So you can see a connection between your lack of exercise and the lethargy you are describing'. Sometimes clients lack correct information about their behaviour, often as a result of the confusing messages they get from the media. This could influence their decision making in a negative way. Therefore, it can be necessary to put right any such incorrect information.

A helpful way of trying to understand all sides of the conflict or ambivalence, is to carry out a decisional balance. This involves exploring with the client the pros and cons of change and the pros and cons of staying the same. This task can be done verbally or, additionally, on paper with a balance sheet. Figure 9.1 shows the layout of a typical balance sheet. Even if done without the use of paper, the matrix should be in the back of the mind of the practitioner to remind them to consider all sides.

The following dialogue demonstrates the technique with someone ambivalent about reducing their chocolate intake. It starts by considering the pros and cons of the current behaviour.

	Advantages	Disadvantages
Change		
No change		

Figure 9.1   Decisional balance sheet.

P: So, what do you like about eating chocolate?

C: I really enjoy the taste.

P: It's really satisfying.

C: Yes, especially when I've had a hard day.

P: You find it helps you wind down.

C: It just balances things out. If I'm feeling a bit yukky then I like to have something nice to make me feel better again.

P: So it helps take your mind off unpleasant feelings.

C: Yes.

P: What else do you like about it?

C: That's it really, it just tastes so nice.

P: What don't you like about it?

C: Well, it's not helping me lose weight.

P: And your weight concerns you.

C: Yeah, I've put on quite a bit lately and I can't fit into some of my clothes.

P: What else bothers you about eating chocolate?

C: I know it's not good for my health, I mean my mum's a diabetic.

P: And you think that your chocolate eating may be taking you that way.

C: Yes.

P: And you wouldn't want that.

C: No definitely not, I know how difficult it is for her.

P: What else?

C: That's all I can think of at the moment.

P: Perhaps I can just summarise where we've got to so far. On the one hand you like eating chocolate because you really enjoy the taste and it helps you avoid unpleasant emotions, and yet you recognise that it's contributing to your weight gain and it isn't benefiting your health. Is that right?

| C: | Yes.

The next section explores the pros and cons of changing behaviour.

| P: | Let's just assume temporarily that you did change and reduced your chocolate intake. How might you be better off?

| C: | Well I know it would be better for me and help stop me getting like my mum.

| P: | It would be good for your health.

| C: | Yeah and I'm sure it would help me lose weight.

| P: | Which sounds as if it is important to you.

| C: | Yes, very.

| P: | What other ways would you benefit?

| C: | I'd feel I could control it. At the moment I can't seem to stop myself. Whenever I see it I just eat it.

| P: | So if you were to stop, you'd feel a real sense of achievement.

| C: | Yes.

| P: | What concerns you about reducing your chocolate intake?

| C: | I'd miss it. That really nice taste.

| P: | The pleasure of the taste.

| C: | Yeah.

| P: | What else concerns you?

| C: | The fact I might not be able to do it.

| P: | What about that possibility concerns you?

| C: | Well if I couldn't control it I'd have to resign myself to the fact that I'll probably always be overweight.

| P: | And you wouldn't want that.

| C: | No definitely not. |

| P: | So, at the moment, you can see that your current chocolate consumption is contributing to your weight gain and may be leading you down the same route as your mother and that if you were to change you'd lose some weight, which is really important to you, and you would feel a sense of achievement in showing yourself you can control it. Yet on the other hand you really enjoy the taste of chocolate and are anxious about trying to change and failing. Is that right or have I missed anything? |

| C: | No that's right, it's so frustrating, I wish there was an easy answer. |

Another way of getting this particular dialogue started is to ask, 'If you did decide to change and reduce your chocolate, in what way would it affect you and how might it affect other people'.

When carrying out this weighing-up process for physical activity it is slightly different because you are encouraging the client to take up a new behaviour as opposed to giving up an existing one. Because of this it is usually not very helpful to ask what they like about their current inactivity. People often look a little confused when asked this, as inactivity isn't thought of as a discrete behaviour in itself. A better way of starting might be, 'I wonder if you could tell me why you think you might need to make a change in the amount of exercise you do'. This should invoke a response such as, 'well if I don't, I'm probably going to end up being even less fit'. This response is a negative aspect of staying the same or not changing, and you can then progress from these.

| P: | What concerns you most about becoming less fit? |

| C: | I might not be able to do certain things. |

| P: | Such as? |

| C: | Well, I might not be able to get up stairs or even walk without getting out of breath. |

| P: | And you wouldn't want that. |

| C: | No way. |

| P: | What else concerns you about your lack of exercise? |

Once you have exhausted the cons of not changing it is better to move over to the change side of the equation because, as mentioned already, if you now ask about what the client likes about not taking exercise they usually struggle to answer. You can come back to this point later. Here is an example:

| P: | If you were to make a change, how would your life be different? |

| C: | I'd be able to get out and about more. |

| P: | And that's something you would enjoy. |

| C: | Yes, I really enjoy walking, particularly with my wife, but I get worn out so easily at the moment. |

| P: | So you'd like to go out walking more yet at the moment you would find that too difficult. |

| C: | Yes, I need to be fitter first. |

| P: | How else would you benefit from taking more exercise? |

| C: | Well, it would stop my wife nagging me to stop moping around at home. |

| P: | Your wife has noticed that you don't exercise much. |

| C: | Yes, she's always reminding me because she's pretty fit. |

| P: | So far then, you think that if you don't start to take a bit more exercise you're probably going to end up really unfit which will stop you getting out very much and may even stop you moving around your own house, and if you can get a bit fitter you'd be able to go out walking more often and further with your wife, which is something you both enjoy. Have I understood you properly so far? |

| C: | Yes. |

| P: | What concerns you about getting fitter and doing some more exercise? |

| C: | I might do too much and have a heart attack. |

| P: | You're worried about not knowing how much you can do. |

| C: | Yes. |

P:	What else might you not like about it?
C:	It's just the effort really. Once I sit down in front of the television I can never motivate myself to get up.
P:	So getting started might involve a bit of discomfort.
C:	Yes, I'm just lazy I suppose.
P:	You don't think right now that you could make the effort even if you wanted to.
C:	Well, no I think I could, I just have to convince myself that it's worth it.
P:	So let me see if I've heard you right. Staying as you are means that you are not putting yourself at risk of a heart attack and means that you don't have to tolerate the discomfort of pulling yourself away from the TV and yet you're concerned that if you don't start to do something you might end up being less able to do some day-to-day things and miss out on walking with your wife which you enjoy and would like to do more of.
C:	Yes, that's it exactly. I don't know what to do for the best.

It is important here not to oversimplify the difficulty of this task. Clients may sometimes be aware of this conflict and still not proceed towards change. However, they probably have not discussed it in this much detail before. When written out like a balance sheet it sometimes appears obvious to the professional what the next step is. This is an easy mistake to make. Do not assume that the values you put on each cost or benefit are the same as the client's. What appears to be one small thing on the cons of change side of the balance may be of utmost importance to the client and sufficient to prevent them from changing. Also, as we observed in the previous dialogue, even when people desperately want to change and can clearly see the benefits, they may still make no effort to do so, believing that success is beyond their grasp.

So merely weighing up the pros and cons may not be sufficient to invoke a change. Once you are confident that you have explored all aspects of the client's ambivalence and summarised them accurately, a useful exercise at this point can be to ask the client how to proceed. Phrases such as 'What do you think the next step is?',

'Where do you think we go from here?' or 'What do you think needs to change?' can encourage the client to become 'unstuck', as they often are stuck at this stage.

If the client answers 'I'm not sure', then it can be helpful to summarise their options. This example follows on from the previous one about chocolate eating.

P: So let's see what your options are. One is, you stay as you are and continue eating the same amount of chocolate, which you said would probably mean more weight gain and possible negative consequences on your health. A second, would be to consider what options there are for changing, which might lead to a lower weight and a sense of achievement if you were successful, or a final option is that you go away and think about it, now that we've had this discussion, and then we could meet in a few weeks to see how you feel then.

C: I think I'd like to consider what I might be able to do to change.

This summarising exercise focuses clients' minds on what the choices are and also helps them see that they are the only ones who can decide what decision to make. As Prochaska (1994) has pointed out , 'the client will only move towards action when they believe that the positive aspects of change outweigh the negative aspects and the negative aspects of staying as they are are greater than the positive ones.'

Working through this can get the client to a point where a decision not to change can take place or a point where they wish to think about it more. Both of these are legitimate conclusions to a consultation. However, with both of them it is important to negotiate a follow-up appointment to encourage the client to continue in the change process. Be careful though, not to appear to put pressure on the client to move too quickly. Try to convey your continued interest in helping the client in any way you can. 'If it's okay with you I'd like to give you a call in a month or so to see how you feel then. Whatever you decide is up to you, no one can decide for you. I'll support you whatever your decision.'

Finally, summing up clients' choices with them can create the transition to the next stage, preparation. Other clues to help you decide whether to move on or not are 'self-motivational' statements made by the client that indicate a commitment to change (Miller 1983). Examples include:

'This is worse than I thought, I must do something about it.'
'I guess the time has come for me to start doing something about this.'
'I do want to change but I'm not sure how to go about it, it all seems so confusing.'
'I've had enough of being like this, I've got to do something about it.'

In summary, this stage is about trying to understand clients' ambivalence and tipping the balance in favour of change. It is important to consider how their current behaviours are affecting them both positively and negatively, assessing the possibility of change and the cost and benefits associated with it. It is also important to consider how clients' lives will be affected if they change successfully. Consideration should be given to how both sides of the balance affect individuals and their environments, including their relationships with others.

Chapter 10
Preparing for Action

Characteristics of the client preparing to change

Clients in the preparation stage have made a commitment to change and are likely to take action in the near future. They are also likely to have had a recent attempt at change. It might seem that this is a relatively easy stage to help clients through; it is merely a case of giving appropriate advice on the best course of action. However, clients in preparation still have some degree of ambivalence. Although they may have decided that it would be better to change than stay as they are, they still don't move into action. Clients may not be able to see a plan of action that they think will work for them or their commitment is contingent on an 'easy' plan being made available. Another possibility is that the barriers to achieving change are so great that the client believes that they are insurmountable. An example might be the case of a single mother who has decided to take part in a regular exercise class but it turns out that the leisure centre offers no childcare facilities.

Some clients in the preparation stage are committed to taking action yet lack the skills to select a suitable plan or lack coping skills for the inevitable difficulties. If such clients are asked what difficulties they anticipate in changing they often respond with comments such as, 'I'm really motivated this time, nothing's going to get in my way, just tell me what I need to do'. Strong intentions to change mixed with poor skills commonly lead to only temporary changes in behaviour.

In summary, clients in the preparation stage have made a commitment to change but are still likely to be somewhat ambivalent about it. They have evaluated the disadvantages of their current behaviour as greater than the advantages, plus the disadvantages of change are now less than the perceived advantages.

Processes emphasised during preparation

Self-liberation, social liberation.

Therapeutic goal of the preparation stage

To help the client explore options for change and to choose the best course of action. To strengthen commitment and confidence for change.

Working with the preparer

As already mentioned at the beginning of this chapter, even though clients appear to have made a decision to change at this stage, they are still likely to be ambivalent. It is important therefore, not to think that the strategies used in the previous chapter for building motivation are now redundant. It is quite likely that you will need to revert back to some of them during this stage to strengthen the client's commitment for change.

There is a major shift during this stage from concentrating on establishing reasons and motivation for change to negotiating a plan for change. Your goal during this stage is to elicit a range of alternatives for change from your client and ultimately a SMART plan. SMART plans are Specific, Measurable, Achievable, Realistic and Time orientated. However, it is not the practitioner's job to prescribe change or tell clients how to change or even to teach clients the skills required for change, but to help the client explore the options for change and determine the course of action they think will work best for them. This is part of the process of social liberation; becoming aware of changes in the environment that may help increase access to the new behaviour, for example becoming aware of the wide range of healthy food choices, or the availability of exercise classes in the evenings.

Equally important at this stage is the process of self-liberation, which is making a commitment to change and believing that change is possible. This means not only exploring the options for change, but deciding on a specific plan for change, and being confident about putting it into action.

Once the client has recognised that the reasons for change outweigh the reasons for staying the same, the first task is to help the client consider what might be done to achieve change. Some useful open-ended questions which help in getting started, and encourage self-responsibility and freedom of choice, include:

'What do you think you will do now that you've decided you'd be better off cutting down on your fat intake?'
'Where do you think we go from here?'
'What do you think the next move is from here?'
'How do you think you might go about changing. What do you think your options are?'

At this point it is quite common for the client to respond thus:

'I don't know, you're the expert, you tell me.'

This is particularly likely to happen when clients are paying for your help. In fact in the exercise field it is very common to hear fitness instructors talk about the exercise prescription, meaning that once the client has indicated a desire to change all they need is instruction on how to change. If this strategy was adopted it would run the risk of undoing all the good work done so far. Instructing the client to carry out a plan that is unacceptable is most likely to be met with resistance and a whole string of reasons why the plan won't work. However, there is also a danger in offering no advice and getting the client to do all the work. You do have expertise in the sense that you know what the options are, what appears to work for other people and what the scientific literature says works and what doesn't. Therefore, it is important to let your client benefit from your expertise while still being client-centred. An example of how to word things when the client asks for direct advice could be as follows:

'Well, it seems that there are a number of things that people have found to work, not just one. What I can do is to tell you what other people have found to be helpful for them. However, at the end of the day, you'll be the best judge of what you think will work for you. Shall we talk about what some of the possibilities are?'

Another important task during this stage is to try to build the client's self-efficacy. Self-efficacy is the belief that one is capable of performing a specific behaviour that will produce a desired outcome. People's self-efficacy will determine their choice to take on a certain behaviour, the amount of effort they will expend and how persistent they are in the face of difficulties. Self-efficacy is influenced by past success in the particular behaviour, observing others successfully perform the behaviour (especially those perceived as similar to oneself), verbal persuasion and the physiological response to a behaviour.

Therefore, individuals who have been successful in the past at performing a given behaviour are more likely to feel more confident about doing it again in the future. This may mean that individuals who are attempting the particular behaviour for the first time may need it broken down into small steps. Being confronted with the final behaviour may seem overwhelming. For example, pointing out to a client that the ideal amount of exercise is 30 minutes a day on at least 5 days per week, may seem so out of reach that the client never even starts. However, introducing 10 minutes a day and gradually increasing by 5 minutes a month may seem more possible.

Seeing other people similar to oneself successfully perform a behaviour is an important factor. This is observed in many forms of groups, such as weight loss groups, smoking cessation groups, Alcoholics Anonymous, exercise to music classes and gyms. In fact, some leisure services departments have capitalised on this idea by running a variety of specialist exercise groups, including over-fifties classes, pre- and post-natal classes, exercise prescription schemes, ladies only mornings, disabled sessions, and dedicated sessions for particular ethnic groups. The idea is that efficacy beliefs will be strengthened by learning new behaviours with like-minded people. However, groups may not be for everyone. It may be sufficient to talk about other similar clients who have been successful in changing their behaviour:

'A lot of the people I see feel anxious like you do. They think that they can't do it, but then are surprised at how quickly they grasp it once they start. In fact, they often tell me they would have tried much earlier if they had known how easy it was going to be. What do you think?'

A client's confidence will also increase when the advice-giver firmly believes that the given behaviour is attainable by the client. Again, if the professional describes the behaviour in terms of small steps that the client believes are achievable then they are more likely to perceive the task as within their capability.

When people become emotionally aroused (anxiety, heavy breathing, palpitations, sweating) during stressful situations they often interpret it as a sign of vulnerability. This then reduces their self-efficacy and their performance is inhibited. When imagining entering an exercise to music class for the first time, clients may find that they feel anxious, their heart rate rises and their breathing increases. They may interpret these responses as evidence that they cannot carry out the behaviour and are likely to avoid going. Avoiding attempting the behaviour is also likely to reinforce the view that the behaviour is unattainable by the client. In other words, 'if I predict that I won't be able to perform the exercise class and that I may make myself look foolish I am likely to evaluate this as quite "terrible". As a result I am likely to feel anxious which will increase my breathing and heart rate. These responses then reinforce my view that something terrible *is* likely to happen, and so I avoid the situation. My avoidance proves to me that I do not have the necessary ability to cope with the difficult situation that I predicted would occur.' Anticipating such situations with clients and talking them through can go a long way to reducing arousal.

One way of starting to build clients' self-efficacy is by showing them how many change options there are. This is encouraging because it means that there isn't only one way of achieving change. If there was, it could seem rather daunting to the client. 'What if I try it and fail? Then I'll never be able to change'. This is another reason to convey to clients that there isn't a 'best' way and that the only 'best' way is the one that they're able to do. If you try what you believe to be the best way and it doesn't work then you are resigned to staying as you are. Putting across a menu of options can also encourage people who have had previous unsuccessful attempts at change. 'I've tried to change before, but I've always slipped back to my old ways.' 'It sounds as if you haven't found a way that works for you yet.'

So to be able to work with people during this stage it is important to be fully aware of the change options for both eating and exercise.

Change options for eating

Because our food supply is now so varied and interesting the change options for a healthy diet are almost endless. There are over 12 000 different food items to choose from on a trip around the supermarket! The bottom line though is that any dietary plan should be nutritionally well-balanced and sustainable in the long term. There are many so-called 'diets' around which are not. Some diets, because they are not nutritionally balanced, recommend the use of vitamin and mineral supplements as a top-up to ensure a complete supply. This should not be routinely necessary and it makes much more sense for people to obtain all their nutrients, including vitamins and minerals, from the source that nature intended – food.

As well as being nutritionally sound it is useful to think of the options for dietary change in terms of the five 'Ps', which will make them suitable for short- and long-term change. The eating plan must be:

- **Practical** – based on everyday foods rather than focusing on special nutritional products or expensive and inaccessible foods.
- **Positive** – stress what can be eaten rather than focusing on what to avoid.
- **Personalised** – tailored according to the individual's physiological needs, which depend on age, gender, activity level and body weight.
- **Palatable** – include foods which are liked by the individual.
- **Possible** – take account of social and economic factors such as family circumstances, working patterns, income and cooking skills.

The system used in this book is based on the National Food Guide, called *The Balance of Good Health* (Gatenby *et al.* 1995, Hunt *et al.* 1995b, Hunt *et al.* 1995c). It is so flexible that it accommodates the needs of everyone, from a six foot three, very thin, very active young male to a five foot tall older woman who is quite overweight and takes no regular exercise. It is also nutritionally complete without including long lists of specific foods which people must eat or must avoid. It shows how a variety of foods, eaten in the right proportions, can mean that people don't have to give up foods that they most enjoy just for the sake of their health.

Fruit and vegetables
Choose a wide variety

Bread, other cereals and potatoes
Eat all types and choose high fibre kinds whenever you can

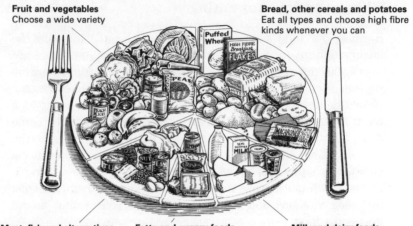

Meat, fish and alternatives
Choose lower fat alternatives whenever you can

Fatty and sugary foods
Try not to eat these too often, and when you do, have small amounts

Milk and dairy foods
Choose lower fat alternatives whenever you can

Figure 10.1 National Food Guide: The Balance of Good Health. (Reproduced with kind permission of the Health Education Authority.)

Although based on the principles of reducing fat (especially saturated fat), reducing sugars, increasing starchy carbohydrate and fibre and reducing salt, the National Food Guide tells its message in food terms, rather than using nutritional language. *The Balance of Good Health* uses a food groups approach because no single food contains all the nutrients in the amounts needed – and no single food is good or bad. However, some are clearly better and some worse than others. A mixture of foods must be eaten in the right proportions, hence the name *The Balance of Good Health.*

The five food groups are:

- bread, other cereals and potatoes;
- fruit and vegetables;
- milk and dairy foods;
- meat, fish and alternatives; and
- fatty and sugary foods.

Figure 10.2 shows the different nutrients which are provided by each group of foods. To get the wide range of nutrients the body needs to remain healthy and function properly, it is important to choose a variety of foods from the first four groups. Foods in the fifth group, fatty and sugary foods, are not essential for health but do add extra choice and palatability. The small proportion of space which this fifth group takes up, which applies to meals and snacks, is reinforced by the verbal message 'try not to eat these foods too often, and when you do, have small amounts'. *The Balance of Good Health* encourages people to eat more fruit and vegetables and more bread, cereal and potatoes than perhaps they do routinely. In fact, foods from these groups should each provide a third of the area on the plate, two-thirds in total.

In reality, the way people could best increase their consumption of foods from these groups would be different. For fruit and vegetables, it is likely that people could eat them more frequently by, for example, having fruit as a snack, having a side salad to accompany a sandwich or having vegetables such as cauliflower or broccoli in addition to the small amount of vegetables in a casserole or stew. Bread, cereals and potatoes may be difficult to eat more often, unless it is by having bread products as snacks, but are probably easier to increase by having larger portions at any one time. This may seem to contradict the old fashioned advice to cut down on such foods. It is now irrefutable, however, that because these foods are filling and not especially high in calories (or fat), unless they are cooked in fat or have butter, margarine or a rich sauce added to them when they are served, they should be encouraged rather than restricted.

The message about the two smaller groups (milk and dairy, and meat, fish and alternatives) is twofold. Firstly, eat slightly smaller portions from these groups than from the fruit and vegetables and bread, cereals and potatoes groups (the model shows that each of these represent about one-sixth of total food intake). Secondly, and perhaps most importantly, choose lower fat alternatives whenever possible.

Inevitably, although clients will find the National Food Guide useful as a starting point, it is likely that they will want specific information about exact quantities and portion sizes, tailor-made for them. There is so much individual variation in nutritional *needs* as well as food preferences, that this is essential for one-to-one dietary advice.

Tailoring advice is not simple. People's needs vary depending on:

The five food groups	Bread, other cereals and potatoes	Fruit and vegetables	Milk and dairy foods	Meat, fish and alternatives	Fatty and sugary foods
What foods are included?	Bread and potatoes are self-explanatory. Bread includes all types of bread. Other cereals means things like breakfast cereals, pasta, rice, oats, noodles, maize, millet and corn meal. Beans and pulses can also be eaten as part of this group.	Fresh, frozen and canned fruit and vegetables and dried fruit. A glass of fruit juice can also contribute. Beans and pulses can also be eaten as part of this group.	Milk, cheese, yoghurt and fromage frais. This group does not include butter, eggs and cream.	Meat, poultry, fish, eggs, nuts, beans and pulses. Meat includes bacon and salami, and meat products such as sausages, beefburgers and paté. These are all relatively high fat choices. Fish includes frozen and canned fish (e.g. sardines and tuna), fish fingers and fish cakes.	Margarine, low fat spread, butter, other spreading fats, cooking oils, oily salad dressings or mayonnaise, cream, chocolate, crisps, biscuits, pastries, cake, puddings, ice-cream, rich sauces and fatty gravies, sweets and sugar.
The main nutrients	Carbohydrate (starch) 'Fibre' (NSP) Some calcium Some iron B vitamins	Vitamin C Carotenes Folates 'Fibre' (NSP) and some carbohydrate	Calcium Protein Vitamin B12 Vitamins A and D	Iron Protein B vitamins, especially B12 Magnesium	Some vitamins and essential fatty acids but also a lot of fat, sugar and salt.

How much to choose	Eat lots	Eat lots	Eat or drink moderate amounts and choose lower fat versions whenever you can.	Eat moderate amounts and choose lower fat versions whenever you can.	Eat sparingly – that is, infrequently and/or in small amounts.
What types to choose	Try to eat wholemeal, wholegrain, brown or high fibre versions where possible. Try to avoid: • having them fried (e.g. chips); • adding too much fat (e.g. thick spread on bread); or • adding rich sauces (e.g. cream/cheese on pasta).	Eat a wide variety of fruit and vegetables. Try to avoid: • adding fat or rich sauces to vegetables (e.g. carrots glazed in butter, roast parsnips); or • adding sugar or syrup to fruit (e.g. stewed apple, chocolate sauce on banana)	Lower fat versions means semi-skimmed or skimmed milk, low fat (0.1% fat) yoghurts or fromage frais and lower fat cheese (e.g. Edam, half-fat Cheddar). Check the amount of fat by looking at the nutrient information on the labels. Compare similar products and choose the lowest.	Lower fat versions means things like meat with the fat cut off, poultry with the skin removed and fish without batter. Cook these foods without added fat. Beans and pulses are good alternatives to meat as they are naturally very low in fat.	Some foods in this group will be eaten every day, but should be kept to small amounts, e.g. margarine, low fat spread, butter, other spreading fats, cooking oils, oily salad dressings or mayonnaise. Other foods from this group really are occasional foods, e.g. cream, chocolate, crisps, biscuits, pastries, cake, puddings, ice-cream, rich sauces, fatty gravies, sweets and sugar.

Figure 10.2 Further explanation of the food groups in the National Food Guide. Adapted from the Health Education Authority's leaflet *The Balance of Good Health – Information for Educators and Communicators.*

1   Gender – women tend to need less energy (calories) than men.
2   Age – older people need less energy than young adults.
3   Being overweight – carrying excess weight means less energy is required to achieve a weight within the healthy range for a person's height.
4   Being very physically active – the more active a person is, the greater their energy needs.

However much total energy an individual requires, the proportion of foods in the diet should remain the same, as shown in the *Balance of Good Health*. Figure 10.3 gives some portion sizes for a range of foods within each of the five food groups, which are adapted from the Health Education Authority's *Changing What*

Food	Daily measures	What counts as a measure?
Bread, other cereal and potatoes	5 to 14	Breakfast cereal – 3 tablespoons Bread/toast – 1 slice Bread bun or roll – $\frac{1}{2}$ Pitta bread or chapati – one small Crackers – 3 Potato or sweet potato – one egg-sized Plantain or green banana – matchbox size
Fruit and vegetables	5 to 9	Vegetables – 2 tablespoons Salad – small mixed Fresh fruit – one piece Stewed or tinned fruit – 2 tablespoons Small fruit juice – 100 ml or $\frac{1}{4}$ pint
Milk and dairy foods	2 to 3	Milk – 200 ml or $\frac{1}{3}$ pint Yoghurt or fromage frais – small pot – 150 grams Cottage cheese – small pot – 100 grams Piece of cheese – matchbox size – 40 grams or $1\frac{1}{2}$ oz
Meat, fish and alternatives	2 to 3	Beef, pork, ham, lamb, liver, kidney Chicken Oily fish } 50–70 grams or 2–3 oz White fish, not in batter – 100–150 grams or 4–6 oz Eggs – 2 (up to 6 per week) Tinned baked beans – 3 tablespoons Dish based on pulses or lentils or dahl – 3 tablespoons Nuts or peanut butter – 2 tablespoons or 60 grams (2 oz)

Food	Daily measures	What counts as a measure?
Fatty and sugary foods	0 to 4	Butter or margarine/spread – 1 teaspoon Low fat spread – 2 teaspoons Cooking oil, lard, dripping or ghee – 1 teaspoon Mayonnaise or oily salad dressing – 1 teaspoon
		All of the following count as one measure per portion:
		fatty bacon sugar (e.g. in drinks) sausages luncheon meat pork pie biscuits sausage roll crisps rich sauce fatty gravy cream cream cheese
Drinks	Aim for 6 to 8 cups/mugs/ glasses daily	Limit intake of sugary drinks and choose sugar free, diet or slimline soft drinks or mixers where possible.
Alcoholic drinks	Up to 21 units a week for women. Up to 28 units a week for men.	One unit is $\frac{1}{2}$ pint of beer/lager/cider, 1 small glass of wine or 1 pub measure of spirits. If you are overweight, bear in mind that alcoholic drinks provide extra calories.

Figure 10.3 Portion sizes (or measures) for a range of foods within each of the five food groups. Adapted from the Health Education Authority's *Changing What You Eat* booklets.

You Eat booklets (Hunt 1995d). Figures 10.4 and 10.5 show how you would work out the nutritional requirements for two different people, one an obese, physically inactive middle-aged man and the other a marginally overweight woman in her late thirties, who is always on the go and wants to make sure she doesn't gain any more weight.

The logic, flexibility and nutritional completeness of *The Balance of Good Health* makes it an ideal tool for use in one-to-one dietary consultations. It provides instant clarity to common questions such as, 'So exactly what is a balanced diet?' and 'What should I eat to be healthy?'

Many of the different dietary methods and techniques available, especially for weight loss, are nutritionally unsafe when compared with the National Food Guide. They are probably ineffective too, certainly in the long term. Any diet which promises a 'quick fix',

Food groups	Number of measure
Bread, other cereal and potato	6
Fruit and vegetables	8
Milk and dairy	2
Meat, fish and alternatives	2
Fatty and sugary foods	1

Figure 10.4   Food group requirements of an obese inactive man in his early fifties.

Food groups	Number of measures
Bread, other cereal and potato	7
Fruit and vegetables	9
Milk and dairy	2
Meat, fish and alternatives	2
Fatty and sugary foods	2

Figure 10.5   Food group requirements of an overweight active woman in her early thirties.

which is what most clients would like, is not worth considering. Physiologically it is neither safe or desirable to lose any more than $1\frac{1}{2}$ to 2 lb or up to 1 kg per week of fat. If people are losing more weight than this it will be lean tissue and water, and it is highly likely that the yo-yo dieting effect will set in. Rapid weight loss is frequently followed by weight gain and the weight regained probably contains more fat than that which was lost. Yes, dieting can make you fat if done too hurriedly.

There are many books around which advocate the 'miracle cure'. As far as we know, none to date has provided the 'magic bullet' which everyone is looking for. Maybe it's time to stop looking and get to grips with the reality that changing what people eat isn't easy but is possible and with a bit of hard work, can have impressive consequences in how people feel, how they look and perhaps most importantly, in improving their health in the long term.

Although it is not possible to go into detail here, for the record it may be helpful to list those diets which we consider are not particularly suitable because they (a) are nutritionally incomplete or unbalanced, (b) cannot be sustained in the long term; or (c) have not been shown to be effective. Few, if any, of these encourage an individual to take full responsibility for a personal dietary plan.

1   Severely limited range of foods, e.g. the egg and grapefruit diet.
2   Non-food, e.g. very low calorie milk shake drinks.
3   Banning certain food, e.g. the no chocolate diet.
4   Encouraging a single food, e.g. the crisp lovers diet.
5   Unbalanced, e.g. unlimited protein and barely any carbohydrate, unlimited meat/fish/chicken and salad/veg/fruit and no bread/pasta/cereal/potato/rice.
6   Food combining. There appears to be nothing especially magical about this despite the claims about enzymes, gut functioning and absorption of nutrients, though the regime does force people to eat a healthy diet. For example, the diet doesn't allow combining fat and carbohydrate at the same meal so automatically excludes popular indulgences like chocolate, cakes, biscuits, puddings, rich sauces and fried foods such as crisps or chips.
7   Rigid meal plans, e.g. pre-set menus which don't account for likes and dislikes or the need to accommodate a person's lifestyle. For example, suggesting poached eggs for Tuesday lunch and liver for dinner is not helpful for someone who works on a building site and hates liver!

Having said that, different things work for different people. Some clients may have success stories of their own, or friends, with some or all of the above. *The Balance of Good Health*, however, is simply a diet for good health with a structure which makes it flexible and simple to understand and easily maintained for life.

Change options for exercise

Change options for exercise break down into four main areas.

1   Frequency – how many times per week.
2   Duration – how long the exercise will be for each session.
3   Intensity – how hard the exercise will be.
4   Mode – what type of exercise, e.g. cycling, walking, weight training, etc.

In 1990 the American College of Sports Medicine published a position statement on the 'recommended quantity and quality of exercise for developing and maintaining cardiorespiratory and muscular fitness in healthy adults' (ACSM 1990). The recommendations included the following.

1 Frequency of exercise: 3–5 days per week.
2 Duration of exercise: 20–60 minutes of continuous aerobic activity.
3 Intensity of exercise: 60–90% of maximum heart rate.
4 Mode of exercise: any activity that uses large muscle groups, can be maintained continuously, and is rhythmical and aerobic in nature, e.g. walking, hiking, running, jogging, swimming, cycling, etc.
5 Resistance training: strength training of moderate intensity. One set of 8–12 repetitions of 8–10 exercises that condition the major muscle groups at least 2 days per week.

The frequency of exercise is most likely to be limited by the client's available time. In the review by Hillsdon *et al.* (1995) the average number of exercise sessions per week at the completion of most programmes was two to three. It is important that clients who can only exercise at this minimum frequency are realistic about the time required to achieve observable benefits. To achieve the energy expenditure associated with reduced morbidity and mortality and to contribute significantly to weight control, the duration and intensity of exercise would need to be long and hard. For most people the risk of injury and the likelihood of dropping out are increased with high intensity exercise (running, high impact aerobics). Therefore, a compromise must be negotiated. This will probably mean an exercise plan which can be continued over a longer duration, as it can more easily be incorporated into current lifestyles, but one where results arrive slower than might be desired. Being honest with clients about what can be expected, means they are less likely to be disappointed.

The duration and intensity of exercise are very much related. Higher intensity activity can only be performed for a short duration, whereas more moderate intensity activity can be tolerated for longer. If the exercise frequency is at a minimum, the duration can be increased to build the total energy expenditure without having to exercise at a very high intensity. Most people, once they have made a decision to exercise on a given day seem happy to spend between 45 and 60 minutes doing so. Moderate intensity exercise is not only associated with a reduced injury and drop out rate, but it is the intensity at which most people naturally exercise, given the choice.

Exercise intensity can be measured a number of ways. It can go from using sophisticated equipment such as telemetry heart rate monitors, which give a constant read-out to the user, manual measurement of the pulse during exercise, or the simple talk test (explained later). Heart rate monitors are expensive and can be an added inconvenience, having to put them on and take them off for every exercise session. They are more suited to athletes and clients who have a high risk for a cardiovascular event, who require more supervision. Both the heart rate monitors and measuring the pulse manually require the calculation of a heart rate range based on 60–90% of maximal heart rate. This assumes that the person's maximum heart rate is known. You will only know this if the client has had a maximal exercise test, or stress test, which is very unlikely. Fortunately, there is a simple formula for estimating maximal heart rate. Deducting the client's age from 220 will give you a reasonable estimate of maximal heart rate which errs on the side of caution. This figure can then be multiplied by 60–90% to produce a range of exercise heart rates. Here is an example for a 35-year-old.

220 – age = 185
60–90% of 195 = 111–167 beats/minute

Most people find it difficult to locate their pulse at rest let alone while exercising. To be accurate, the heart rate needs to be measured within 10 seconds of stopping exercise. If not, the heart rate measured will be an underestimate of the actual exercise heart rate and may result in the client deciding to increase the exercise intensity which may be dangerous. This method should therefore be used with caution. A more simple method is the talk test. The talk test means that while exercising someone is breathing quite heavily but could still hold a conversation, albeit with a little difficulty, but they would not have enough air to sing. If they are so out of breath that they can no longer converse with anyone, then they should slow down. This simple method is sufficient for most apparently healthy adults.

For those individuals who really aspire to high levels of fitness, perhaps for a particular sport, it will be necessary to exercise at a higher intensity. Before this is encouraged, consideration should be given to the risk status of the individual. Guidelines for establishing safety will be discussed later. However, it is worth noting at this point that if there is any doubt as to the safety of exercise for an individual, then medical advice should be sought.

When discussing the intensity of exercise with clients it may be simpler to refer to exercise as either light, moderate or vigorous. These descriptions translate approximately to 35–59%, 50–74% and 75%+ of maximum heart rate respectively. Examples of activities that generally fall within these categories are shown in Table 10.1.

Table 10.1   Light, moderate and vigorous activities (adapted from the Allied Dunbar National Fitness Survey).

Light	Moderate	Vigorous
Table tennis, golf, social dancing (if not out of breath or sweaty)	Swimming, football, tennis, aerobics, cycling (if not out of breath or sweaty)	Squash
		Running
		Football
Bowls	Table tennis	Swimming, tennis, aerobics, cycling (if out of breath or sweaty)
Fishing	Golf	
Darts	Social dancing (if out of breath and sweaty)	
Light gardening	Heavy DIY	
Light DIY	Heavy gardening	
Slow walking	Heavy housework	
	Brisk walking	

If the frequency, duration and intensity of exercise are similar then the mode of exercise is less important. As described above, any aerobic exercise (exercise which requires oxygen) that uses large muscle groups and is rhythmical may be used. This means the options are wide ranging. Clients can choose from something as simple as brisk walking to joining a gym or exercise class.

It can be seen that there are many possible combinations within these recommendations. These recommendations are somewhat different from the ones mentioned in Part I, which were recommendations for health. The research discussed in Part I shows that it may not be necessary to perform the same quantity and quality of exercise required for 'fitness' to attain health-related benefits. Table 10.2 compares the two sets of recommendations.

Although there are differences, the health recommendations can be incorporated into those for fitness. The recommendations for health emphasise the frequency and duration of exercise more so than the intensity. In other words, they suggest exercising at the lowest intensity, at the highest frequency and for at least half the duration of the fitness recommendations. For beginners and non-athletic adults, lower intensity activity is recommended because it is associated with a lower risk of injury and less drop-out.

How the variables above are used will depend on what benefits the client is aiming to achieve. If health or weight loss are the most motivating factors then the recommendations for health will be sufficient, but if the benefits required are more aligned to fitness then the fitness recommendations should be followed.

Discussions with clients about the exercise plan should involve each of the variables described above, with the end result being a clear plan of action. We have found it useful to have each of the variables written down. This helps to make it clear to the client how they all fit together.

Table 10.2   Comparison of exercise recommendations.

Variable	Fitness	Health
Frequency	3–5 days per week	Most, preferably all days of the week
Duration	20–60 minutes continuously	At least 30 minutes that can be accumulated in bouts of no less than 3
Intensity	60–90% maximum heart rate	At least moderate intensity
Mode	Any activity that is aerobic in nature	Not specified, but brisk walking given as a common example
Resistance training	8–12 repetitions of 8–10 exercises at least 2 days per week	None specified

Barriers to change

As you consider each of the options when dealing with a client in the preparation stage, they should be asked about what the likely outcome would be if they adopted that particular option. For example:

'What do you think would happen if you did try that option?'
'How do you think that would turn out, if you did do that?'
'How do you think that might work?'

As you go through this process clients are likely to raise difficulties in implementing each of the options. Such difficulties might be described *as barriers to change*. The barriers they anticipate may reduce their confidence in successfully implementing the plan and prevent them from initiating change. Therefore, it is important to discuss them and not just brush over them. Some common external barriers for both exercise and eating are listed below, with examples of how clients may express their concern.

Eating

- Skills: 'If I'm honest I don't really know how to cook'.
- Facilities: 'I don't have a microwave oven or a wok and storage space for fresh fruit and veg or frozen vegetables is very limited'.
- Financial priorities: 'I find it difficult to afford all the fruit and special low fat things you need for a healthy diet'.
- Food likes: 'I just don't really like a lot of healthy foods, never have done. For example the only fruit I'll eat is bananas, I hate all vegetables and I'm not fond of fish'.
- Time: 'I just seem to be rushing around all the time. I never have time to chop all those vegetables and cook proper food'.

Exercise

- Poor access to facilities: 'I rely on public transport and it takes about an hour just to get to the centre'.
- Financial priorities: 'If I need to buy any special equipment I won't be able to do it, I just can't afford it'.

- Weather: 'I like the idea of brisk walking, but what about when it's raining?'.
- Physical limitations: 'I'm not sure I'll be able to do much. I've always had pains in my knees when I exercise much'.
- Time: 'I work such late hours, I never have the time to fit in an hour's exercise'.

Overcoming the barriers

Although being described here within the 'Preparing for Change' chapter, it will be clear by now that some barriers will probably have already occurred at other stages and will probably occur again in future stages in the change cycle. Some have already been discussed in the 'Contemplation' chapter. The nature of the barriers are usually different at the different stages:

- Contemplators: see barriers as reasons for not changing.
- Preparers: anticipate the barriers which may be associated with the specific plan they are considering.
- Those taking action: may experience small and specific difficulties associated with their plan as they start to implement it, which they didn't anticipate and with which they now need help.
- Those in maintenance: may experience new difficulties associated with the ongoing effort required to sustain change or with external factors which have changed. They may also dislike the way they, themselves, have changed as a result of the changed behaviour, which they disapprove of.

Care is required, however, not to slip into expert mode and prescribe specific strategies on the 'how tos' of overcoming some of these obstacles. The onus is on the client to try and solve such difficulties:

'I can see how it would be difficult if that happened. You'd have to work quite hard to find a way round it.'
'It sounds as if that could be a problem. How do you think you might overcome that, should it occur?'

Responding to the barriers which clients raise should involve a combination of careful listening, accurate reflection, and open questions about possible solutions. Being genuine and empathic is especially vital at this point. Having got this far the whole therapeutic alliance could crumble if the client gets a feeling that you think any of the barriers are unreal, easily surmountable or simply 'excuses'. What follows is an example of discussing potential barriers with a client in the preparing to change stage.

P: So what people or things might get in the way of your new eating plans?

C: Well, I keep thinking about how unhelpful my husband has been in the past. He just doesn't understand that this is so important to me. Because I'm not overweight or anything he just can't see that I have to keep an eye on my diet. He tries to tempt me all the time and sometimes my will power just cracks.

P: So you haven't found him very supportive before.

C: No not at all. But this time it might be better. He knows I need to get my blood cholesterol level down. I keep saying it'll be the death of me.

P: So it's in the interest of your health.

C: Yes. But I really need his support. I think I'll suggest we sit down and have a serious talk through all this tonight.

P: OK. That sounds as though it's important to you. Perhaps we can discuss how you get on when we next meet? Is there anything else which worries you about not keeping to your plan?

C: Just me really. I'm afraid I don't have much will power. I might give in when I think about the foods I'm missing or if someone offers me them.

P: So you might veer off your plan sometimes but you do still feel it's important to get your cholesterol level down.

C: Oh yes most definitely.

P: OK. I can see that. So what particular kind of situations do you imagine might make it difficult?

C: Well ... eating out, celebrations ... or the kids tucking into chocolate cake or something.

P:	So shall we focus first on eating out.
C:	Uh huh.
P:	What could go wrong?
C:	Everything! Other people are choosing all the kinds of things I'd like but can't have, it all smells so delicious and it's especially hard when I'm so hungry beforehand that I just go mad. And the others try to tempt me, you know. 'Go on, have a dessert, just this once won't hurt'.
P:	Yes, I can imagine that would be very difficult. Let me check that – it's the smell, that you're hungry, that others can choose differently and they make you give in? I wonder which of those you could plan ahead for?
C:	Well, I suppose I could just avoid eating out altogether though that seems a bit extreme! I could always have a light snack a couple of hours before going out, just a couple of crackers or something, just to take the edge off my appetite so I'm not ravenous when I come to choose from the menu.
P:	Great idea. Anything else?
C:	Well you've got me thinking about my friends. Maybe, like my husband, they just don't understand how important this is. I could have a bit of a pep-talk with them on the 'phone beforehand. That way they won't go on, just understand that I'm choosing the fruit salad or asking for no butter on the veg because of this cholesterol thing.
P:	I can see that might help ...

So you can see how helpful it is, to break the perceived barriers down into the specific elements of the problem, and ask incisive questions to encourage the client to come up with some solutions. This way the client feels valued, you're not suggesting that her concerns aren't real and you genuinely care enough to help her come up with her own answers. She also gains confidence in her belief that she can succeed.

Once you have been through each option with the client, it will probably be quite clear which of the options appears to be a favourite. This will probably be the one that raises the least potential obstacles and also the one that they express the most confidence about. At this point it is necessary to discuss the plan in more detail to arrive at a SMART plan.

Sometimes, when going through options for change with clients, they may appear to be favouring an option that could be harmful or is very unlikely to lead to the outcome they were hoping for. On these occasions you have a responsibility to make clients aware of your concerns without reducing their freedom of choice:

'As I've mentioned before, how you go about making changes is your choice. However, I want you to know that I'm concerned about the choice you seem to be considering. If I might, I'd like to tell you why I'm concerned.'

Your concern might include eating plans that are not nutritionally balanced or exercise intentions that may not be safe for the client to do. This may be because of existing health problems the client may have. Appendix C shows how to establish the safety of exercise for clients.

Once the client appears to have decided on a suitable plan, encourage the client's self-responsibility by asking for information as to how the plan might be implemented:

'What might stand in the way of your good intentions?'
'And if that happened, what might you do to work round it?'
'How do you think you might get started?'
'What steps do you think you need to take to put this plan into action?'
'How do you think you will be able to do that?'

It may also be helpful to find out if other people may be able to help or hinder the plan:

'Is there anyone who could help you with that, or get in the way?'

Also, it is important to examine clients' expectations regarding the time it may take to achieve their goals. A mismatch in expectations and reality is likely to result in disappointing and a reluctance to continue with change strategies. This is frequently a problem with weight loss when clients wish to lose 4–5 lbs or more per week (see Chapter 14 for discussions on realistic weight loss goals). Although there are no hard rules about the amount of behaviour change that will produce certain outcomes, it is possible to make reasonable estimates.

Developing an action plan

The following examples are just two ways of developing a plan of action for changing exercise and eating behaviour in collaboration with the client.

Exercise

P: So you seem to be clear that taking regular exercise will help you play more games with your son and not leave you so out of breath every time you use any stairs, and yet you are concerned that exercise requires a lot of hard work which you're not sure you'll be able to do.

C: Yes, those things are really important to me now. I've got to start doing something about it before it's too late.

P: Where do you think we go from here?

C: I suppose I ought to think about what I need to do.

P: What do you think your options are?

C: I'm not sure, as you know I've never done any exercise before, and I really don't fancy running. What do you think?

P: Well the good news is that there isn't one best way of taking exercise. What I can do is to tell you what some of the options are. We can then discuss each of them and you can consider which, if any, you think might work for you, remembering that you can always come back and try another option if it doesn't work for you. What do you think?

C: Yes, that sounds good. So I don't have to go running?

P: No. Perhaps I can show you what choices there are and then we can discuss them.

C: Okay.

P: With any exercise the things that need to be considered are what type of exercise of activity you will do, how often you are going to do it, in other words how many times per week, how long will be spent doing it on each occasion and how much effort or exertion it will require. Perhaps we could start with the first of these. Have you given any thought to how many times per week you might do some physical activity?

C: I know I could definitely do two sessions, maybe three. ‹

P: What about the length of each of those sessions? How long are you prepared to spend each time?

C: I suppose, I ought to do half an hour at least, probably nearer an hour.

P: Let's assume you chose to do two 60-minute sessions a week, how would that work out?

C: If I make the decision to do some exercise on any particular day, I want my effort to be worthwhile, so I think I will do an hour. Yes, I could do that.

P: What about the difficulty of each of those hour long sessions?

C: Well if it's too hard I won't be able to do it and I'll quickly give up, but I want to feel I've done something.

P: I wonder if I can offer you some advice here.

C: Uh-huh.

P: Most people find exercising for about an hour that they could do moderate exercise but not vigorous. Moderate exercise is sufficient enough difficulty to help you towards the benefits you described.

C: But how will I know if I'm doing moderate?

P: A good indicator is what's called the talk test. That is, when you are exercising it shouldn't be so hard that you couldn't talk to anyone and yet it should be hard enough that you will have some difficulty carrying on a conversation without pausing for breath. What do you think about that?

C: That sounds easy enough, but I wouldn't be able to do that if I was running.

P: Well, running is regarded as a vigorous activity, it is much harder work and isn't something to start with right away. Examples of moderate intensity activities include brisk walking, leisurely swimming, cycling for pleasure, recreational tennis, doubles badminton or non-competitive singles. Anything that is the equivalent of brisk walking for you can be classified as moderate. Which of these do you think might work for you?

C: Well I like to walk anyway, but I normally go quite slowly. You know, more of a stroll.

P: So how do you feel about converting that to more of a march?

C: I think I could do that.

P: It sounds as if you're finding something that could work for you.

C: Yes, I feel confident about what we've discussed so far.

P: So what do you think the first step is, what do you think you need to do to get started?

C: I think it's just a case of deciding what days I can fit these walks into. I can definitely do one on a Sunday. I often like to walk on a Sunday morning anyway. If I could break the other hour up, I mean do half an hour before work and another after work, I could do that.

P: That sounds great. Where would you do that?

C: I could walk to the train station instead of driving and then walk home again in the evening. It would be good to do that in the middle of the week because I am normally carrying more on Mondays and Fridays. So I think I will do it on Wednesday.

P: So let's just summarise what we've covered so far. You think that you could do one 60-minute walk on a Sunday and on Wednesdays you will walk 30 minutes to the station in the morning and 30 minutes home in the evening.

C: Yes, that sounds okay.

P: How do you think these changes fit in with your goal of being able to run round with your son more and becoming less out of breath after walking up stairs?

| C: | Well, I think it's a start, it's certainly more than I'm doing now. I know that if I could go more regularly it would be better, but I'll see how it goes. I don't want to say I'll do something I can't stick to. |

| P: | You seem to have thought this through and you appear to have come up with something that you are confident about doing. Do you think you are ready to do this? |

| C: | Yes, definitely. |

| P: | Thinking about the next few weeks, is there anything that might interfere with your plan? |

| C: | I don't think so, only if it rains the whole time I suppose. |

| P: | And if that was to happen, what might you do then? |

| C: | Well, it's not that big a problem, I can easily carry a small umbrella in my work bag, and at weekends I've got one of those big golf umbrellas. In fact, it might be quite nice walking in the rain as long as I know I can go home to a nice hot shower and a cup of tea. It'll probably be refreshing. |

| P: | Have you any questions at this stage? |

| C: | No. |

| P: | When do you think you will start? |

| C: | This week, yes Wednesday. |

| P: | That's great. When do you think we should meet again? |

| C: | I'd like to see you in about a month if that's okay. |

| P: | Sure. |

Eating

Here's how you might introduce the National Food Guide as a framework within which your client can consider their options for changing diet.

| P: | So now you've made the decision, how do you think you might go about changing what you eat? |

C: I'm really relying on you to advise me about that. What do you think is the best thing for me?

P: Well different things seem to work for different people. I do have a general system which all patients use differently. It works better for some than others, it's very flexible. We could try that for starters and within the overall system you can judge what particular changes would suit you best. Would you like to hear a bit about it?

C: Yes I'll give it a go.

P: (Describes the five food groups system and the proportions which make up a healthy balance. Discusses broadly what amounts would be suitable for someone of the client's age, gender, weight and activity level.) So, how do you think this model might work for you?

C: Well it makes quite a lot of sense really. I can see straight away that I don't eat nearly enough fruit and vegetables. I could easily eat more.

P: OK. So how would you go about that?

C: Well I could have a banana sliced on my breakfast cereal which is what my wife tends to do. I could easily take an apple or orange to eat at work and ... well, I suppose I would quite enjoy an extra serving of veg. with my main meal. It would definitely be more filling then.

P: Great, so that's three more extra fruit and veg. servings a day. What about any of the other food groups?

C: Well, this fatty and sugary group seems really small for all the different things in it. But I don't think I could give up my bag of crisps every day.

P: No problem. Are there any other changes you might consider in that group?

C: Biscuits and cake are in this section aren't they?

P: Yes.

C: Well, I tend to go for those things just for the sake of it really, not because I'm hungry. I'd be prepared to cut the biscuits out.

P: Altogether.

C: Well, maybe not completely, but definitely during the week. Say 5 days out of 7.

P: Uh hum. OK. I wonder, does anything jump out at you from the other groups?

C: I must say I noticed how relatively small the meat and the dairy sections are. I'm wondering if I eat too much meat and cheese.

P: OK, but notice there are some alternatives.

C: Oh I see, so fish and beans are in the meat group too? Well that would be OK. I'll give up the meat now and again for fish. Would that be helpful?

P: Yes, sure. How often do you think you could do that?

C: I love fish actually so I'd have that a couple of times a week, but without the batter of course! I'm rather partial to baked beans as well. Is that the kind of beans this means? Beans on toast is always a nice change.

P: Quite! That's just what it means. So you have the beans instead of meat?

C: Yes. And I won't be surprised if you say my pork pies are banned!

P: Well, nothing's ever banned. But you're right, pork pies are very high in fat. What might you have instead?

C: Well I tend to grab one at the service station if I'm on the road at lunch time but it's just a habit really. I could just as easily have a sandwich. I notice that the section with bread in is huge. Is that really right, that I could have 9 servings of bread a day?

P: You could if you wanted to. Or you could swap some for other starchy foods like potatoes or pasta or rice. Or breakfast cereals come to that.

C: That's amazing ... I'd never have thought I could eat so much ... though I suppose it's good for filling you up?

And so it continues, with discussion about as many changes as the client wants to consider. The final stages and ending the session will go something like this.

P: So it sounds as though you have quite a little list of things to tackle.

C: Yes but it's not nearly as daunting as I thought. I had it in my mind I was going to be on crispbreads and raw carrots from now on!

P: So you're quite pleased. Shall we sum up what you're going to do?

C: Yeah, remind me what I've let myself in for!

P: Well from what I recall, you're going to:

- have more fruit and veg – three more lots a day;
- aim for nine lots of 'bread, cereal and potato', for example by eating sandwiches at lunch instead of pork pie;
- have fish twice a week instead of meat;
- have baked beans once a week instead of meat; and
- cut down the biscuits to weekends only, but you will stay on the crisps.

How does that fit with what you remember?

C: That's exactly right. Not so bad really is it?

P: No and it sounds as though you really think you can do it. So what steps are you going to take to get this plan into action?

C: Well I do need to restock the freezer and change my shopping habits a bit I suppose. Get some fruit in a bowl at the office too. I could ask them if they would put fruit out at meetings as well as biscuits.

P: OK. And what might jeopardise your plan?

C: Mmm. Well ... I do eat out quite a lot. That can be difficult. And because the kids never seem to stop eating there are always biscuits around the house which could be tempting.

P: So eating out regularly sounds as thought it may present problems.

C: It could but to be honest most restaurants have decent fish so I could choose that, or perhaps even go for a vegetarian choice now and again.

P: Yes, to get your beans! And what about the biscuits?

C: It's a case of keeping them hidden away really. If I don't see them I don't get tempted. Maybe I can talk to the kids and ask them to hide the biscuits in a cupboard.

P: Sounds helpful. Now I notice that we're running out of time so we do need to end today's session. Have I left you feeling unclear about any of the changes?

C: No I don't think so. It will probably soak in a bit better when I have read through the booklet at home though.

P: Yes. And if you have any specific queries, do telephone. I'm here every day except Friday and a good time to get me is between 9.00 and 9.30 in the morning before I start seeing clients. If you can't get through you can always leave a message for me to call you back.

C: Thanks. It does make a difference knowing I can get hold of you. There might well be a few things I find I'm not clear on once I get home.

P: OK. So shall we meet again in a month's time, as we discussed, to see how it's going?

C: Yeah, that would be useful.

P: Great. So you can make your appointment with the receptionist on your way out. Cheerio for now.

In this dialogue, the client, having been given a general framework, came up with most of the changes himself. In doing so he felt more confident in his success because all of the changes seemed reasonable. Having thought about any difficulties in changing he came up with his own solutions. By asking the right questions in the right way at the right time, in this case, the practitioner had to give very little factual information apart from the initial explanation about the food groups system. In addition, by letting the client know exactly when and how to contact her, her offer of support was perceived as genuine.

Summary

On completion of your discussions about the action plan, it is beneficial to summarise the final plan. Some people also like to write this down and give it to clients. The summary might include: (a) the reasons why the changes are important, including the benefits they will bring, (b) what changes are going to be made; (c) what steps will be taken to implement the plan; (d) how other people may be able to help; (e) what may get in the way of the plan and what will be done if things do get in the way; (f) how they will know if the plan is working, and finally (g) how they are going to reward themselves if it is successful. An example of a standard form of summarising the final plan is shown in Appendix D.

Chapter 11
Taking Action

Characteristics of the client taking action

Clients in the action stage are taking their first tentative steps towards change. Their temptations to return to the old behaviour and their self-efficacy (task specific confidence) are delicately poised, reflecting the high rate of relapse during this stage. Clients increasingly rely on support from others during this difficult stage, seeking reassurance about their decision to change, to increase their self-efficacy and as an external monitor for their progress. The use of behavioural processes is particularly important during this stage. It requires clients to have a degree of competency in applying these processes and to work hard. Success or lack of it at this stage can be influenced by the immediate consequences of the behaviour. Clients still have some unresolved ambivalence at this stage and if the immediate consequences of change meet their worst fears then action can be short lived.

If clients go into the action stage hoping for quick success they can often be disappointed. Typically, the results of changes in eating and exercise behaviour take longer to see than a lot of clients are prepared to wait for. Positive reinforcement about change and encouraging clients to attribute change to their own efforts are important tasks during action.

In summary, clients in action are starting to implement their action plan and are experiencing the immediate consequences of change. As changes occur, clients will constantly be reappraising the pros and cons of change.

Processes emphasised during action

Counter-conditioning, stimulus control, helping relationships, reinforcement management.

Therapeutic goal of the action stage

To help clients increase their self-efficacy, focusing on successful changes and helping them attribute such changes to their efforts. To help develop strategies for coping with stimuli that can lead to a return to the old behaviour. To offer support and reinforce convictions towards longer term change.

Working with those taking action

There is a fundamental shift in strategies during this stage. Until now the processes emphasised have been experiential, focusing on building and strengthening motivation to change. Now that the client has started to implement his plan, the focus shifts to more behavioural processes aimed at keeping the plan on track. The processes emphasised during this stage are aimed at altering the environment to reduce the likelihood of unhelpful behaviours or to increase the likelihood of a helping behaviour occurring. The processes are stimulus control, counter-conditioning and reinforcement.

Stimulus control

Stimulus control involves changing the environment to reduce the number of prompts or cues to return to the old behaviour, or increasing prompts and cues for the new behaviour. Examples of modifying stimuli include:

- Removing all calorie-dense and low-nutritional-value foods such as biscuits, chocolates, cakes and crisps, etc., from the home.
- Buying only healthy, less calorie foods from the supermarket.
- Choosing a route to walk home that doesn't involve passing a confectioners or bakers, or not walking down the ice cream isle at the supermarket.
- Making social plans to avoid being at home alone.
- Taking up interesting activities to reduce the likelihood of becoming bored when home alone.
- Meeting friends at the gym or leisure centre, not the pub.
- Not watching TV immediately on arriving home.

With exercise behaviour it may be more useful to increase positive cues for exercise rather than reduce cues for sedentary behaviour. A good example of this occurs during the summer, when many people take up tennis each year during the Wimbledon tournament. Other examples of cues to increase exercise and also some to increase healthy eating might include:

- Always keeping some workout kit in the car.
- Writing each week's workouts in a diary.
- Having someone call you to remind you to be at the gym at a certain time.
- Driving home via an exercise facility or park.
- Meeting other people to take part in exercise, perhaps joining a tennis club, athletics club, softball team, tea dancing club, etc.
- Having fruit around the house and office.
- Socialising at restaurants with healthy menus (perhaps vegetarian or fish restaurants).
- Ordering healthy sandwiches for the office a week in advance to reduce spur of the moment decisions.

The practitioner's aim is to help clients control cues for their own behaviour. This will involve helping them to reduce cues for the undesirable behaviour and increase cues for the new behaviour. Sometimes clients have difficulty identifying the cues and prompts for their behaviour. On such occasions it can be helpful for them to complete a diary or log book, often referred to as self-monitoring (Appendix E). The aim of the exercise is for clients to learn what people, events, places or feelings trigger their eating or exercise behaviour. Once these triggers have been identified the task would then be one of reducing the cues for the old behaviour and increasing the cues for the new behaviour. Self-monitoring has consistently been associated with improved short-term adherence to behaviour change.

Counter-conditioning

Counter-conditioning is learning to respond differently to stimuli or cues that normally lead to troublesome behaviour. That is, when we are unable to avoid cues for the old behaviour and are exposed to them, we learn to respond in a new more constructive way that does not lead to a return to the old behaviour. For example, we may learn to look at chocolate biscuits, imagine how nice they taste, experience the urge to eat them and then go without. It is common for people to be so conditioned to this stimuli that they suggest that they were 'out of control' or 'just couldn't stop themselves'. Sometimes learning to respond differently to such stimuli may involve engaging in some other activity, such as taking some exercise or doing some cleaning. In other words, distracting oneself from the stimulus.

Counter-conditioning may also involve gradual exposure to a stimulus and learning to respond differently. For example, clients may gradually increase the length of time they expose themselves to their favourite food without eating it and tolerating the discomfort associated with going without. Each time they do this successfully their confidence increases and the discomfort they experience reduces. A good example of this is when people first go without sugar in their tea. Initially they find the taste unpleasant, but they force themselves to continue. Eventually, as time goes by, they find they enjoy the taste of tea without sugar, and in fact now actually dislike the taste of tea with sugar in it.

In summary, counter-conditioning involves having a plan to respond to various cues and prompts in a way that does not lead to a return to the old behaviour. Examples might include:

● Planning strategies for eating out with friends such as choosing in advance or suggesting an alternative restaurant which has healthier options.
● Doing some exercise, doing some housework, or engaging in some hobby or pastime whenever the urge to eat something sweet arises.
● Learning to say no to friends who always offer you a sweet at restaurants.
● Practising relaxation exercises when stressed.
● Varying the exercise routine when it becomes boring.
● Learning new low fat recipes when food becomes boring.

Reinforcement management

Reinforcement management aims to increase the frequency of the desired behaviour as a result of its positive consequences. The consequences of a change in behaviour can be regarded as reinforcing if they increase the frequency of the desired behaviour or punishing if they decrease the frequency of the desired behaviour. If, when a client first takes up running, they feel good and relaxed when they have finished, they are more likely to want to run again than if they felt nauseous and light headed. Reinforcement can be both positive or negative, both resulting in increases in the desired behaviour. Positive reinforcement, as the name might suggest, results from the consequences of engaging in the new behaviour being interpreted by the individual as pleasant or positive. Positive reinforcement can come from a variety of sources:

- Observation from the client that they are making progress towards their goal; losing weight, getting fitter, reduced lipid levels, reduced blood pressure, etc.
- Approval from others; comments such as 'you're looking good', 'haven't you lost some weight' or 'I see you are up to 3 miles on that treadmill'.
- Praise, reinforcement, encouragement and support from the practitioner.
- Increase in positive emotions such as happiness and pleasure.

The role of the practitioner in providing positive social reinforcement should not be underestimated. Genuine encouragement and support from a professional have consistently been shown to assist the acquisition of new behaviours and support the maintenance of existing behaviours. This is particularly important when people have slipped back from behaviours that involved the support of others. When people stop attending groups for behaviour change, such as exercise classes or weight loss classes, they not only experience the loss of not continuing with the new behaviour but they also lose the social contact and support from other group members. During this time the practice nurse, doctor or exercise professional can be a very important source of support and encouragement.

As described, having encouragement to hand, especially at the times when things seem difficult for the client, is a real boost at this stage. Examples might include:

- Letting a close and trusted colleague know about your eating or exercise plan so that they can not only avoid inadvertently putting temptations in your way, but also show interest by asking how it's going.

- Talking to your partner about how important your diet or exercise plan is so that they can give appropriate, regular support and reassurance and be available for you when the going gets tough.
- Letting your children know that you're taking on a new way of eating so that they can help in two ways: indirectly, for example by preparing their own snack after school to avoid you having to be tempted; and directly, for example by expressing a genuine interest in your progress and offering encouragement.

Negative reinforcement is not the same as punishment. Negative reinforcement involves an increase in the frequency of the new behaviour because the new behaviour reduces existing negative states. Examples include:

- Reduction in depression or low mood.
- Less negative comment from others, perhaps resulting from a loss of weight.
- Less breathlessness or physical discomfort when carrying out day-to-day tasks.
- Reduction in stress.
- Less tiredness and fatigue.

Punishment, used to decrease the frequency of the old less desirable behaviour, is much less effective than reinforcement of the new behaviour. The main reason is that punishment often results in negative emotions such as guilt, hurt and anxiety. Such negative emotions tend not to lead to constructive appraisal of what led to the slip or lapse, but typically lead to an increase in the old behaviour.

Changing the frequency of a behaviour by altering its consequences is sometimes referred to as *contingency management*. Contingency management is a type of reinforcement and involves rewarding oneself with positive reinforcement, contingent on performing a specific behaviour. For example, clients may allow themselves to sit down and watch television each day only when they have completed a one mile walk. Watching TV is the incentive for them to carry out the walk. Written contracts between practitioners and clients are often used to motivate clients to perform agreed upon behaviours. Contracts with clients, if used, should include the following:

- A clear description of the behaviour.
- Duration and frequency of the behaviour.
- Clearly defined positive reinforcements for successful completion of the behaviour.
- A means of accurately monitoring the behaviour.

Not surprisingly, during the early part of action there are many cues or temptations to return to the old behaviour, sometimes referred to as high risk situations. The professional can help clients identify such cues and use the processes described above to help them either avoid the temptation altogether or learn to respond to it constructively. During the first follow-up session, a few weeks into action, it is common for clients to describe events which they found difficult and where they may not have been able to adhere to their intentions. The role of the professional during these sessions is to assess how well the behavioural processes are being applied and provide assistance when errors in the use of the processes are being made. Clients' successes to date should be put down to their own efforts in an attempt to improve their self-efficacy. When clients successfully employ the processes described above, they are more likely to evaluate themselves in a positive way and will have increased confidence for coping with future prompts and cues to return to the old behaviour. Examples of situations that present a temptation to return to the old behaviour for eating and exercise, where the behavioural processes will need to be applied, are listed below. These are not all of the possible scenarios but are some of those commonly presented by clients.

Eating

- Restaurants: 'It was difficult when we went out for a meal at my favourite restaurant. I couldn't help choosing what I always have there, spare ribs and chips with garlic bread followed by cheesecake.'
- Appealing shops: 'When I'm walking past that bakery which makes the best flapjack and custard slices in town, it's torture!'.
- Shopping for the basics: 'I try not to go shopping when I'm hungry but I get tempted when there are so many things, none of them on my list of course, on special offer'.
- Limited choice: 'It's not easy working in a catering department

where staff are entitled to free meals. There's only ever the pie and chips left'.

- Partners: 'My partner's not supportive because she just doesn't have the same motivation to do it' or 'She just adores cooking and experiments with new (not healthy) recipes to show how much she cares about me. How can I cope with that?' or 'She loves me and says she prefers me the way I am'.
- Parents and other family members: 'We're going to stay with his parents for the weekend and they always prepare delicious home baked food. They're irresistible and his mum would be so offended if I said no'.
- Eating companions: 'What about my colleague who I usually eat lunch with? He's very skinny and always has a very large, very high fat cooked meal at midday, with pudding and custard. It's so hard when he does that'.
- Celebrations: 'I suppose life is full of special occasions like birthdays, wedding anniversaries and all that. I shouldn't complain but I really don't know how I'm going to avoid indulgences then' or 'But the two week summer holiday/ Christmas is coming soon. That's bound to be difficult'.
- Times: 'My weak time is around 5 in the afternoon when it's a couple of hours before dinner and I'm always peckish. I have a habit of nipping in to the newsagents at the end of the road for some chocolate'.
- Mood: 'I know that whenever I feel a bit low I turn to my favourite biscuits to make me feel better' or 'When I've had a bad day I eat to cheer myself up'.
- Energy: 'I know that when I get really tired I'm tempted to eat all the wrong things'.

Exercise

- Energy: 'I'm really tired after a day at the office. I can't think of anything else but going home and putting my feet up' or 'I start thinking about the effort of riding that bike and immediately then start thinking about putting it off until tomorrow'.
- Partners: 'I never see you these days, you're always off at the gym'.
- Friends: 'Why don't you come down the pub tonight after work? One night away from the gym won't hurt you' or 'You never come out any more, you're becoming a real bore'.

- Boredom: 'Sometimes I find exercise really boring and so I think of things I'd sooner be doing'.
- Weather: 'I started off all right, but then it rained for a week and I didn't do anything'.
- Frustration: 'I thought I'd notice some differences by now, but I haven't'.

All of the above situations are not uncommon. Learning to cope with such situations and with others is a fundamental part of long-term success in behaviour change.

Summary

Although strategies for coping should not be imposed on, or prescribed to, clients, the practitioner may help clients to consider counter-conditioning, stimulus control and reinforcement strategies. As mentioned in the previous chapter care should be taken not to slip into expert mode and proceed to resolve clients' problems for them. The onus is on the client to try and solve such difficulties. The practitioner can suggest strategies that appear to help 'some people' sustain change in the first few weeks and months but the client will be the one to decide how to implement such strategies. This is especially the case with reinforcement management. What might appear to be rewarding for the practitioner can be seen as a punishment for the client. One other point of caution with reinforcement, especially when trying to change eating behaviour, is to avoid using food as a reward.

During the action stage, the client is likely to experience a whole range of emotions and consequences as a result of making changes in behaviour that can be very stressful. For this reason, it is important for the practitioner or a significant other to be available for support and understanding. Reassurances about the decision to change will be sought quite often, especially from the practitioner who will probably be seen as someone that can be trusted and cares about the client.

The following dialogue is an example of how to negotiate such processes while still being person centred.

P: Perhaps you could tell me about how you've been getting on since we last met a month ago.

C: Generally very well. I've managed to get to the gym about three times each week, which is what I said I would do.

P: You sound really pleased. You set yourself quite a tough task, what with all the other commitments you have. You've worked hard to fit it all in.

C: Yes, on the whole I'm pleased. I am a bit concerned about what's been happening this last week though.

P: Do you want to tell me a bit about that?

C: Well, a couple of times this week I've planned to go to the gym and thought, ah to hell with it I'd sooner be at home with my feet up.

P: And then...

C: I didn't go, I went straight home.

P: How did you feel about that?

C: I felt really bad. I didn't enjoy being at home any earlier, I just kept thinking I should be at the gym. I'd been doing so well up to then.

P: So, it sounds as if you've been pleased with what you did up to that point, but you're a bit disappointed with this last week.

C: Yeah, I don't want to undo all the good work I've done so far. I mean I'm already starting to feel the benefit.

P: Are you saying that you want to find a way of getting round this?

C: Yes, definitely.

P: I wonder if you've thought about ways in which you could do things differently should you find yourself in this situation again.

C: The thing is not to ponder on it for too long. Once I get in the car and start driving to the gym, I'm fine. And I enjoy it when I get there. It's just making the first move.

P: It sounds like you're saying that the longer you think about going home the more likely you are to choose that option.

C: Yeah.

P: What do you think you might be able to do to take your mind off it?

C: Uum. Well I did think about writing myself a note to stick on my desk.

P: Saying...

C: Saying that everyday I go home without going to the gym is another day I am further away from getting fit.

P: So, reminding yourself of what might happen if you don't do it.

C: Exactly.

P: What else might you do to increase the probability that you choose the gym and not home when you think about going home?

C: Well, I've got chatting to this chap at the gym. We seem to get on, you know, and he goes at roughly the same time as me. I wondered if I might actually arrange to meet him at a specific time. That way I'd have to ring him and cancel if I went home, and I wouldn't want to do that.

P: That sounds like a good idea. When do you think you might see him?

C: Tomorrow hopefully.

P: So do you think you might approach him tomorrow and explain you'd like his help?

C: Yes.

P: Can we just take a moment to see where we are?

C: Yes.

P: So far you've said that things have been going well up until this week, when you started thinking about going home instead of to the gym. On a couple of occasions you did go home and felt bad because you thought you should be at the gym. You also said that you want to find a way round this so that you can continue and you suggested a couple of things to help you choose the gym when you start thinking about going home. Firstly you said that you could stick a note on your desk reminding yourself of the consequences of not going to the gym and secondly you said that you would ask if you could arrange to meet a person you met at the gym with the idea that breaking the appointment will discourage you from not going. Is that right, or have I missed anything?

C: No, that's exactly right.

P: Assuming that on occasions you might still choose to go home, what might you do to make that a less attractive option on an on-going basis.

C: Normally, the first thing I do is to stick the television on. Then I don't move until I want something to eat. I suppose I could go without the tv for an hour and make myself do some chores that I tend to let build up.

P: You don't sound too convinced.

C: No, I'm just thinking how much I'd dislike doing that.

P: Enough to make you want to go to the gym instead.

C: The more I think about it yes.

P: So, along with the other two things how do you feel about carrying on?

C: Yes, good. I think they'll help. If I can get to the gym even when I feel like going straight home from work, I'll feel really good and more confident.

P: When do you think we should meet again?

C: I'd like to see you again in another month.

P: Okay, well done. You've worked hard and seem to have found ways to overcome potential obstacles. I'll see you then. Just make an appointment at reception.

In summary, this stage is about building clients' confidence and skills for continued behaviour change. This is partly reflected in their ability to apply the behavioural processes associated with this stage to modify the stimuli that might lead them to relapse. Positive reinforcement from the practitioner, along with helping clients attribute change to their own efforts, are important practitioner roles in moving clients towards maintenance.

Chapter 12
Maintaining Change

Characteristics of the client in maintenance

Clients in the maintenance stage are working to consolidate and progress the changes they have made during action. They are actively trying to avoid or prevent 'slips' or 'lapses'. Successful maintainers look out for situations that lead to relapse and develop coping strategies before the situation arises. Others may become exposed to unexpected temptations or urges without a pre-prepared or rehearsed plan and get caught off guard, increasing the likelihood of a lapse. Some clients in maintenance become frustrated at the on-going effort required to sustain changes and gradually over time slip back towards their old ways.

The positive benefits of change for some clients can be so great that the temptations of old are very low and confidence for continued success is very high. These clients are likely to develop the new behaviour as a habit and view the old behaviour in the same light as they previously considered the new one. In other words they are in termination or precontemplation for the old behaviour. Other clients, especially those with perfectionist tendencies, become stuck in the maintenance stage. Although they may continue to display successful changes, they are always anxious about the possibility of relapse and, in their eyes, failure. For these clients, temptations to return to the old behaviour can stay for a lifetime.

Most clients, however, stay in maintenance for at least 6 to 12 months before they no longer really fear relapse. Although they may have temporary slips back to the old behaviour they are likely to achieve long-term changes.

Maintenance also involves clients re-evaluating themselves. The continued application of the behavioural processes developed during action is more likely to occur if clients believe that they have changed in ways which they value. For example, if clients have found that since they have reduced the amount of their favourite foods they eat they have become much more irritable, and this is not how they like to see themselves, they are unlikely to commit much time or effort to further application of the behavioural processes.

In summary, maintenance is about avoiding relapses by learning to cope with and manage difficult situations, and to re-evaluate the kind of person one is, having changed a particular behaviour.

Processes emphasised during maintenance

Stimulus control, counter-conditioning, reinforcement management, relapse prevention strategies, helping relationships plus self-liberation and self re-evaluation.

Therapeutic goal of the maintenance stage

To help the client consolidate changes achieved in action. To identify and develop strategies for dealing with high risk situations to reduce and prevent relapse. To increase self-efficacy towards on-going change.

Working with the client in maintenance

Preparing clients to move from action to maintenance involves assessment of the situations that may result in unhelpful ways of responding to cues and prompts for the old behaviour. This will include assessment of relapse-provoking situations and of the client's alternatives for coping with such situations. Successful maintenance means actively using the behavioural processes of stimulus control, counter-conditioning and reinforcement as well as the processes of self-liberation and self-evaluation. The aim of assessing situations that provide temptation to relapse and developing coping strategies for such situations, is to help build the client's self-efficacy. That is, developing their confidence for dealing with specific relapse-provoking situations. High self-efficacy is a strong predictor of success in coping with such situations and therefore on-going success.

Common cues for relapse include negative emotions such as anger, anxiety and depression, attending social functions, social pressure, craving and frustration. Work carried out by Marlatt and Gordon (1985) suggests that exposure to such situations without adequate coping skills effects self-efficacy and increases the probability of a slip (a temporary return to the old behaviour), followed by a complete return to the old behaviour. These researchers have developed a model of relapse prevention to help explain the process and develop techniques for relapse prevention.

According to the model, relapse starts with a 'high risk situation', that is, a situation that presents a strong temptation to return to the old behaviour. Exposure to a high risk situation without a pre-rehearsed coping strategy leads to low self-efficacy and positive thoughts about the effect of the old behaviour. In the case of food, an example would be being confronted with your favourite, but high fat food, perhaps chips, not having a coping strategy and imagining how very nice the food would be. What follows is an initial slip, or in this case, eating the chips. At this point, once a slip has occurred, clients often perceive a lack of control, resulting in what Marlatt and Gordon (1985) describe as the abstinence violation effect. This is the belief a person holds that once abstinence is broken, complete relapse is inevitable. In eating this is often expressed as 'blowing the diet': 'That's it, I've blown it now, I might as well carry on. I'll start the programme again next week'.

Learning to control slips and preventing them from becoming relapses will be dealt with in the next chapter. For this chapter we will concentrate on the first part of the model which is concerned with preventing the initial slip or lapse.

The relapse prevention model helps us to understand what practitioners can do in supporting a client's decision to change, and providing strategies for recognising and coping with high risk situations in the context of a helping relationship.

The first task requires identifying potential high risk or tempting situations. One exercise for doing this has sometimes been referred to as 'relapse fantasies'. This involves having the client fantasise about future situations that could potentially lead to relapse. Sometimes clients have difficulties with this, particular if at this moment in time they are feeling confident about their abilities. This confidence can sometimes lead to carelessness with the need to apply the behavioural processes to high risk situations. This can result in unpredicted exposure to a high risk situation and relapse.

When people have difficulty in predicting high risk situations it can be useful to draw on previous experience of lapses and relapses.

'During your previous attempts at changing your eating, in what kind of situations did you find it difficult to restrict your fat intake ... and how likely do you think it is that such a situation will arise again?'

At this stage it is better just to list the high risk situations, rather than try and resolve them with your client as they report them. The reason is that the situations given will vary in how likely they are to occur. Therefore, it is probably more helpful for the client to work on situations that are more likely to occur during the next few weeks and months rather than situations much further away.

'So, we've now got a list of situations that you've described could present quite a risk for returning to your old behaviour. Perhaps what we could do now is rank these in order of priority, dealing first with the ones you are most concerned about.'

Once the list has been established and prioritised, it is a matter of working through each item and developing a coping response. As always, this should be done collaboratively with the client, and should not be prescriptive. The first task in going through the list is to gather more details about each of the high risk situations. 'What is it about that situation that is a cue or prompt to eat or not take exercise?' It may not be having chocolate in the house that is the risk, it may be the urge to eat chocolate at certain times of the day or following a stressful situation that presents the greatest risk. It is important to establish a very clear picture of the events leading up to the client's slip or lapse. It may help to imagine that you are a film maker and you are drawing a story board of each of the scenes.

The next step is to discuss with the client what might reasonably be done about each of the situations. This will involve the use of the behavioural processes of stimulus control, counter-conditioning and reinforcement, as described in the previous chapter. As was the case during the preparation stage, there will be a range of strategies for coping with each situation, rather than one 'best' one. This is important, as hopefully it will increase clients' beliefs that they have some control over the high risk situations they find themselves in. If only one coping strategy is available and it does not work, clients are far more likely to attribute their lack of success to some inherent weakness and feel helpless. The feeling of helplessness is unlikely to lead to efforts to explore other coping strategies, and more likely to provoke resignation to the idea that one is not capable of changing under any conditions. However, when people attribute their failure to a poor choice of strategy, rather than some personal weakness, they may well be disappointed, but are more likely to make efforts towards identifying a more effective coping strategy.

Any strategies negotiated with clients should involve the following:

- recognising cues and prompts for the old behaviour;
- avoiding temptations (stimulus control);
- learning alternative coping skills (counter-conditioning); and
- realising the rewards of change (reinforcement).

These skills have been described in the chapter on action. These should be built on and continued during maintenance.

Successfully maintaining a new lifestyle which does not include favourite, high fat or calorie dense foods (or at least far less than one is used to), or now includes regular exercise, demands a significant re-ordering of priorities and a re-evaluation of oneself. As already mentioned, this requires continued use of the behavioural processes. Perhaps most important in all of these is self re-evaluation, because if a person does not believe that maintaining change results in them viewing themselves more positively, then application of the behavioural processes will not be performed with much conviction.

Self re-evaluation involves a reassessment of the meaning and place of the behaviour in the person's life. This process is very important during contemplation, as discussed in Chapter 9, where it includes:

- an increase in negative feelings or emotions about the existing behaviour being considered for change;
- an increase in positive thoughts about self-control;
- increased self-confidence; and
- thoughts about a reduction in the problems associated with the old behaviour.

During maintenance, the same evaluation takes place, but for the new behaviour, including:

- an increase in positive feelings and emotions about the new behaviour;
- positive thoughts about continued self-control; and
- increased self-efficacy and an awareness of the rewards of continuing with the new behaviour.

The task for practitioners in applying this process involves helping the client to: review the changes that have taken place since adopting the new behaviour; consider how the behaviour has affected them personally as well as others involved in their lives; and evaluate the changes as either positive or negative.

When clients believe that they are becoming more of the person they would like to be, and at least one significant other person reinforces this belief, they are more likely to experience positive emotions about maintaining change, feel more confident about their ability to cope with high risk situations and acknowledge the rewards associated with the new behaviour. For example, most people regard exercise as a 'good' thing to do, whereas they may regard drug taking as a 'bag' thing to do. Also, people are more likely to think of themselves as being 'good' if they engage in 'good' behaviours.

Most people would like to think of themselves as good rather than bad and would also like others to view them this way. People who take part in regular exercise often report increased feelings of confidence, self-mastery, competence and higher self-esteem, feelings valued highly by most people. Therefore, if changing from being a sedentary person to an active person is seen as doing something 'good', and as a result people feel more confident, and have a sense of accomplishment and competence (feelings they value), then they are more likely to continue to work at main-tenance.

However, if people who exercise are considered to be vain, show-offs and obsessive (qualities people don't value) and as a result of changing people feel more irritable, worn out and have less time with their family (more things they don't value), then people are unlikely to continue to work at maintenance.

The self re-evaluation process will also involve clients thinking about the possibility of relapse and evaluating the meaning of relapse for them. As a result, it is not uncommon for people in maintenance to live with feelings of dread and anxiety about the possibility of relapse. This might sound surprising since the person has successfully engaged in a new behaviour for at least 6 months. However, in spite of this apparent success in adopting and maintaining a new behaviour, temptations for relapse are still relatively high and confidence in coping with high risk situations low. The low confidence for coping with temptation, even after a significant period of successfully doing so, is often a result of anxiety. Anxiety arises from being overly concerned about the possibility of a future event which, if it occurred, would be described as terrible or awful by the person and would, in their mind, reveal them as weak and inadequate.

With exercise and eating, people are anxious about the possibility of relapsing back to a sedentary lifestyle or to overeating. They normally infer that this would mean that they have failed in their attempt to change and evaluate failing as terrible and proof that they are weak. When people feel anxious they tend to overestimate the threat of the situation and underestimate their ability to cope with it. They then avoid or withdraw from the threat, in this case a high risk situation for relapse. Feeling anxious and avoiding high risk situations prevents people from developing and practising new coping strategies for dealing with such situations. Although avoiding situations that might lead to relapse may work some of the time, it would be unrealistic to think that such situations could be avoided all of the time.

This means that there will be times when a person is exposed to a high risk situation without a strategy or any skills for coping with it. As we have already said, exposure to high risk situations without a coping strategy is more likely to lead to a slip and a reduction in self-efficacy. In addition to avoiding or withdrawing from anxiety-provoking situations, people often attempt to obtain short-term relief from the discomfort of the anxiety itself. With eating this can often be self-defeating.

For example, a man may be anxious about the possibility of giving in to urges to eat his favourite high fat food. He then attends a party, where to his horror, he is offered that food. His anxiety goes up as he contemplates the possibility of eating the food which, in his mind, would prove how weak he is. The anxiety itself is uncomfortable and he wishes to avoid the discomfort. He has learned that for him, the best way to remove the discomfort of anxiety is with food, and he eats. So, in spite of feeling anxious about relapsing and eating what he said he wouldn't, the anxiety increases the likelihood of relapsing rather than reducing it.

When people feel anxious at the possibility of relapse it is often because not only have they rated their success or failure at coping with a high risk situation, but they have also rated 'themselves' as people based on their behaviour. For example, if a woman sets herself the goal of not eating dessert at dinner, but then gives in to her urges and eats the dessert, she would conclude that she had failed at avoiding dessert at dinner, which proves that she is a failure. When people conclude that not only did they fail at the task but they personally are failures because of it, they normally also predict that they will never be successful ever again. This rating of our whole self on the basis of our behaviour can easily occur during the process of self re-evaluation.

When people are weighing up the pros and cons of the new behaviour, they can easily use this information to rate themselves. So it can be seen that if people rate themselves according to how well or how badly they performed a given behaviour, rather than just the behaviour itself, then it is no wonder they remain anxious about the prospect of relapse. If on the other hand they only rate relapse as how well or how badly they performed a particular behaviour and don't interpret that rating as meaning anything about them as a whole person, then they are more likely to feel concerned rather than anxious. Feeling concerned as opposed to anxious is a healthier emotion as it helps people to view the prospect of relapse more realistically, and allow them to make a more realistic assessment of their ability to cope with a relapse-provoking situation and deal with the situation more constructively.

To reduce the possibility of clients feeling anxious about relapse, it is important to help them make the distinction between rating their behaviour and rating themselves as a result of their behaviour. An example may help to demonstrate how this may be done:

C: I'm so hopeless, I just can't seem to stop eating chocolate. Everything else I do really well at. I've cut down on other high fat foods, reduced my alcohol and I exercise regularly. It's just the chocolate. What kind of a person can't even say no to a piece of chocolate. I have to spend my whole life avoiding it so that I don't get the urge to eat it. I know we talked about how I might cope when I get the urge to eat it, but I seem to forget that when I get a craving. I just get all panicky, because I know I shouldn't be eating it.

P: You've done so well in so many areas and yet you seem to be frustrated about your lack of success with the chocolate eating.

C: Yes, I'm hopeless with that.

P: When you say, you're hopeless, do you mean that you have been hopeless at resisting the urge to eat chocolate or you are a hopeless person because you haven't been able to resist the urge to eat chocolate.

C: The second one.

P: If your aim is still to find a way to cope with your urges to eat chocolate without actually giving in to them, how helpful do you think it is to rate yourself as hopeless.

C: Not very.

P: Why do you think that is?

C: Well, if I'm really hopeless there's no point in even trying. Which if I'm honest is what I'm doing now. I've sort of resigned myself to the idea that I can't do it, but then I get angry because I think if I can manage the other things okay, why can't I do this?

P: So you can see how rating yourself as a hopeless person isn't helping you at all.

C: Yes.

P: What do you think you could tell yourself about your lack of success with resisting chocolate that might be more helpful to you?

C: I don't know really.

P: One thing you might try is only evaluating your behaviour. So you might say, 'I didn't do very well at avoiding that chocolate tonight. I wish I could've done better, but I didn't, that's too bad. I'm bound to make some mistakes with something that is difficult, but it doesn't prove that I'm completely hopeless. I'm human and humans make mistakes. Now, how can I do better next time?' How does that sound?

C: | Better.

P: | Do you understand why?

C: | Well, it just sticks to the facts.

P: | That's right, because if you were to conclude that 'because I didn't resist the urge to eat chocolate when I said I would, that proves that I'm hopeless', that would be going way beyond what actually happened. And, when you do that you normally don't consider ways of doing better next time. If you were going to give yourself a single rating, such as hopeless, you'd have to consider all the behaviours you've ever done to be fair to yourself and then you'd have to keep doing it because every minute of every day you perform another behaviour. Can you see how unrealistic that is?

C: | Yes, definitely.

P: | It is perfectly reasonable to rate how well you do at any given behaviour, because that helps you decide what you might need to be differently to improve for next time. However, every time you go beyond rating the behaviour and rate yourself as well, you're always going to feel anxious at every possibility of performing less than perfectly.

C: | Yes, I can see that. So, what can we do about the chocolate?

P: | Perhaps we can consider what other coping strategies you might use when you get the urge to eat chocolate.

C: | Yes, okay.

Clients who have had a number of unsuccessful attempts at changing their behaviour are quite likely to interpret this as some personal weakness, rather than them having not yet found a copying strategy that works for them. This is particularly likely with clients who don't develop a repertoire of coping skills, but rely on will power. Most people regard willpower as their ability to apply effort and determination to a given task. However, will power alone is not sufficient for effective action. Just being more determined and working harder can end up making this more difficult. Although determination is necessary, without the necessary behavioural skill it can be misdirected. It is like trying to undo a nut on the wheel of a car without knowing which may it turns. Lots of effort and determination in the wrong direction will make it even tighter to undo.

If clients depend on will power alone and are unsuccessful, they are more likely to view themselves as weak and inadequate and are not likely to put their lack of success down to the poor choice of process or coping strategy. This reinforces the idea that clients will tend to do better when they have prepared well for maintenance and developed a range of strategies and skills for dealing with a variety of high risk situations.

In summary, the maintenance stage is an opportunity to review clients' progress to date, including the good things and less good things about changing, and to help them prepare for longer term maintenance. An important point to convey to clients is that it is they who have made all of the changes so far and they who have worked through many difficult and tempting situations.

Chapter 13

When Maintenance Fails

Characteristics of the client who has relapsed

As pointed out before, the most common, although not inevitable, outcome of an attempt to change eating or exercise behaviour, is relapse. Relapse usually occurs as a result of a slip, that is a return to the old behaviour, and can be viewed as a process by which people move back to an earlier stage. Longitudinal data on smokers suggest that most relapsers return to contemplation, with only approximately 15% returning to precontemplation (Prochaska & DiClemente 1984). So, many people who relapse consider making another attempt at change.

Which stage of change clients return to will be strongly influenced by their interpretation of the relapse and how they feel about it. Some may immediately return to action, realising that their return to the old behaviour was only temporary and need not interfere with their longer term plan of permanent change. In fact, they may use this experience as a lesson for future difficulties. Others may experience a sense of failure and feel guilty and frustrated about their inability to change. This can easily lead to low self-confidence about future change attempts. This more negative reaction is more likely to lead to a longer return to the old behaviour.

On some occasions relapse can be intended or planned. For example, people who exercise regularly may choose to rest while on holiday and take no formal exercise, but intend to go back to their normal routine immediately on return.

Processes emphasised during relapse

Helping relationships.

Goal of working with clients who have relapsed

To help the client re-enter the change cycle and take action more effectively on the next occasion.

Working with the client who has relapsed

In the previous chapter we considered how to prepare clients for high risk situations that might lead to a return to the old undesired behaviour. We learnt that confronting a high risk situation armed with a set of coping strategies was more likely to lead to a better outcome than being without such strategies. At this stage, clients have been unsuccessful at coping with a high risk situation and have either slipped or completely relapsed back to the old behaviour.

It is important to make the distinction between a slip and a relapse. A slip is a temporary return to the problem behaviour that may just involve one single episode, such as over-indulging in food at a party or missing an exercise session. A slip can lead to relapse but is unlikely to be the sole cause. Relapse is a complete return to the problematic behaviour. Working with those who have slipped and trying to prevent a relapse involves different skills from those required for working with someone who has relapsed. Therefore these two situations will be treated differently in this chapter.

The relapse prevention model that we introduced in the previous chapter helps increase understanding about what turns a slip into a relapse and how to avoid it. When people slip from a voluntary change in behaviour, a common psychological reaction tends to occur. Marlatt & Gordon (1985) have referred to the reaction as the abstinence violation effect (AVE). This refers to how people respond to breaking a self-imposed rule of abstinence, such as planning to go without chocolate for a fixed period of time. In other words, a person makes a commitment to going without something, such as certain foods, cigarettes or alcohol, for a fixed or indefinite period of time. During this time they experience a slip. The AVE is a reaction to the slip that influences the probability of returning completely to the old behaviour, or a relapse. The AVE can be viewed as a continuum. The greater the AVE the greater the probability of a relapse. There are two main components to the AVE. The first is one where the individual asks themselves why the slip occurs and attempts to identify the cause, while the second is their emotional response to the perceived cause.

When the cause of the slip is attributed to an internal cause, such as a personal weakness or lack of will power, the person feels guilty and in conflict. Also, depending on the extent to which people blame some inherent weakness for the slip, they will feel powerless to regain control of their behaviour. When there is a perceived loss of control there will be a reduction in self-efficacy. This self-blame and the resulting emotions leads to an increase in the AVE and an increase in the probability of a relapse. However, if the cause of the slip is attributed to external factors, such as a temporary lapse in coping with a particular high risk situation, then the AVE will be low, the person will maintain a sense of control and self-efficacy will be stable.

When clients subscribe to the former cause, they feel guilty for breaking their personal rule of abstinence. When people feel guilty because they have done something they believe they absolutely should not have done, they frequently have other distorted thoughts that are likely to lead to a relapse. These include:

- *Over-generalising:* viewing the slip as evidence of complete failure and total relapse. This in turn increases the probability of future slips in the same and other situations. 'That's it I've blown it, I'm off the diet now, I'll never be able to do this.'
- *Selective abstraction:* focusing excessively on the one recent failure and dismissing other successful experiences as having no importance.
- *Excessive responsibility:* when the person assumes all responsibility for failures and uses them as evidence of personal weakness and misses the opportunity to learn from mistakes.
- *Catastrophising:* exaggerating how bad the slip is and instead of taking the opportunity to learn from the slip the person focuses on the worst possible outcome. 'I just won't be able to stop now, this is the trigger to eat and eat and eat. I'll be fat forever.'

Attributing the cause of a slip to personal weakness also focuses people's thinking on themselves, particularly on how they view themselves. Prior to the slip they may have viewed themselves as someone who abstains from chocolate or as an 'exerciser'. Now their behaviour is in conflict with this view since they are eating chocolate or not exercising. This conflict and accompanying guilt are particularly unpleasant. Most people would prefer to relieve themselves of this discomfort. Therefore, the discomfort can act as motivation to further resort to the old behaviour. For dieters, food or particular sorts of foods may have been used previously to reduce negative feelings such as guilt. Therefore, eating, so called comfort eating, can act as a form of negative reinforcement, helping the client escape from uncomfortable negative emotions. To add to this, the immediate gratification of the food can precipitate further unwanted behaviour. Focusing on the pleasure of the immediate gratification can mask the delayed negative consequences of the original slip.

When the AVE is intense people typically have poor expectations about coping with high risk situations in the future. Not only do they have poor expectations about coping with similar situations, but also with any high risk situations and for the foreseeable future. Their view of themselves as weak and lacking in will power makes for little optimism.

It can be seen how important it is for clients not to internalise the cause of a slip. This is highly likely to result in relapse and poor predictions about additional future attempts at change. So how can practitioners help clients to attribute their slip to external factors that they can control?

When trying to help someone who has slipped, the first practitioner task is to make some kind of assessment of the slip. Usually, this involves some retrospective verbal report from the client. The aim of this assessment is to establish how the client sees the cause of the slip. However, this can be difficult as the client may be motivated to avoid being truthful. If the client attributed the cause of the slip to some personal weakness at the time it would have provoked strong negative emotions such as guilt. Questions about the client's attributions are likely to evoke the same feelings of guilt as well as shame perhaps. Clients may attempt to give answers that 'save face' or protect them from feelings of shame and guilt, rather than revealing personal weaknesses. In other words they are likely to attribute the cause of their slip to something external such as stress or social pressure.

This happens more often the longer it has been since the slip. For this reason, it is useful to ask the client to recall a recent event. This will only be possible if the client is seen shortly after a slip. This should be something that is agreed upon at an earlier stage as it is not uncommon for clients who feel guilty about slipping to avoid seeing a professional. When practitioners probe for explanations as to the cause of the slip clients may be somewhat defensive. It is uncomfortable for them to reveal personal weaknesses, and an immediate reaction to threats of discomfort is to protect themselves from it.

There are a number of strategies that can help overcome this problem. Firstly, it might be better to get the client to imagine someone else in the situation and ask them to provide possible explanations as to the possible causes of the slip. People often use different rules for themselves than those they use for others. For example:

| P: | Imagine if it was somebody else in that situation and they had gone straight home instead of exercising. What possible explanations might there be as to why they did that? |

| C: | They might have been tired, they might have known that something they wanted to watch on the TV was going to be on, they didn't stop to think about how important the exercise was or they just don't have much will power. |

| P: | So there could be a number of reasons, some to do with planning or being prepared perhaps and some to do with the person's personality? |

| C: | Yes. |

| P: | Which one of those do you think best explains what happened to this person? |

| C: | They probably just didn't have much will power, the others are just excuses really. |

| P: | And which of those reasons do you think best explains your slip? |

| C: | I suppose the same if I'm honest. I never seem to be able to do things that require much effort? |

It can be seen how de-personalising the slip in the first instance may reveal the client's true thoughts. However, this will not always work and practitioners will need to be wary of clients misleading them. If it does become apparent that clients believe that their slip is proof of some inherent weakness or lack of will power it is important to help them reframe this view to stop a full relapse. Developing and practising the use of coping strategies is a skill and needs to be learnt. As with any learning, mistakes will be made. If clients are taught that behaviour change is a learning process then slips can be viewed as mistakes in the learning process. These mistakes are opportunities to learn, not evidence of complete failure. When viewed this way clients can be helped to see mistakes or slips as a perfectly normal part of the change process. If people never make mistakes how can they learn from them? Clients can be taught that few if any people master new skills at the first attempt. The mistakes along the way provide information essential for long-term success.

Another useful way to view slips is as a one-off decision taken in a difficult situation. Many clients believe that their slip just happened, they didn't choose whether to exercise or not, or whether to eat or not, it just happened. It is important to help clients see that they still had voluntary control over their limbs and that they made a choice. It is important for them to see this as it can help them realise that they are not powerless or out of control in such situations. This needs to be done sensitively though, as clients may sense that you are blaming them for making a bad choice. It is important to show them that you understand why they made the choice they did, while reinforcing the idea that it was in fact a choice.

P: When you say that you were out of control, what prevented you from stopping?

C: I just couldn't. I'd had one mouthful and then I couldn't stop.

P: What do you think would have happened if you had stopped?

C: It would have been horrible. Once I've started I have to finish it.

P: Just for a moment I want you to imagine something. Imagine that I've got your whole family and am holding them to ransom. If you don't stop eating the ice cream I'm going to kill them all. Could you stop?

C: Yes of course.

| P: | Surely if you were out of control you couldn't stop. |

| C: | Well it depends what the circumstances are. When it's that kind of choice you can do it. |

| P: | So it is a choice then. |

| C: | Only when you put it like that. |

| P: | Can you see how you made a choice before. |

| C: | I'm not sure. |

| P: | Well, you had a choice to eat the ice cream or not. From what you've said so far, you chose between the immediate pleasure of the taste and the discomfort you predicted would occur if you went without. What do you make of that? |

| C: | I see what you mean now. |

By creating a situation where the choice is more obvious it is possible to demonstrate to the client that they do have choice and therefore control over a situation.

Trying to get the client to attribute the cause of their slip to more external factors requires a detailed examination of the slip. Things to consider are the difficulty of the high risk situation, the use of an appropriate coping strategy (if any), and other factors that may have influenced the amount of effort put in, such as fatigue, high stress, etc. The aim of this examination is to try and isolate external factors that the client has some control over. External factors can be controlled using techniques such as reinforcement management, stimulus control and counter-conditioning. Once you have examined the slip, you can offer your interpretation of its cause.

| P: | You've suggested that your slip provides evidence that you lack willpower. After listening to what you have said I have an alternative explanation as to the cause of the slip. Would you be interested in hearing it? |

| C: | Sure. |

By asking permission to share your view it doesn't appear that you are just dismissing the client's view. Once you have given your view, you can ask the client what they make of it and whether or not they agree with it.

Having established the cause of the client's slip, it is necessary to re-establish how ready he or she is to explore strategies for dealing with future ones. Once it is clear that the client wishes to continue, the next job is to brainstorm options for coping better with the same situation should it occur again. This should be done in a client-centred way as described in the previous chapters. As a slip can easily lead to a relapse, the time immediately following a slip is a particularly dangerous one. The strategies that you discuss with your client should consider this period. Marlett and Gordon (1986) think of these as 'emergency procedures'. They suggest drawing up a reminder card for clients to carry with them in the event that a slip occurs. Although this should be an individual process. they do make some recommendations, which include:

- Seeing the slip as a warning sign that danger is ahead and action is needed. Try and stop and refer to the reminder card.
- Take a few moments to gather yourself and be calm. Let the AVE pass including the normal immediate feelings of guilt and shame. Remind yourself that a slip is a mistake and is a normal part of learning to change.
- Remind yourself why you are committed to making this change. This single slip doesn't undo all the good work so far.
- Try not to blame yourself. Look at the situations leading up to the slip and look at what you could have done differently. What coping strategies did you have prepared?
- Immediately make renewed plans for coping with this situation in the future.
- Perhaps most importantly, ask for help. Call your practice nurse or fitness professional, etc.

After you have discussed future coping strategies with your clients, rehearse them. Talk through, slowly, the high risk situation and what they are going to do at each stage. Almost like a slow motion fire drill.

Sometimes you will see clients some time after the slip, when the slip led to a relapse. It would be inappropriate on these occasions to immediately try and evaluate what led to the relapse. First, it is necessary to re-evaluate the client's motivation to make another attempt at change. This means going back and using some of the processes discussed in the contemplation stage, and weighing up the pros and cons of change.

However, the person who has been successful at changing for a while and is contemplating another change attempt, is different from the contemplator who has not yet attempted action. The person who has had some success brings to the weighing up process some valuable information about what change means. They have first-hand experience of the consequences of change, both good and bad. The first-time contemplator can only predict what these might be. In addition, the person with some experience of change has developed some coping skills that work. Although these skills were not sufficient, they are useful for the next attempt.

People who relapse do so for different reasons, such as social situations, negative emotions or stress. It is also likely that people relapse for different reasons depending on the point from which they relapsed. It is likely that people who relapse after only a few weeks of action relapse for different reasons than those who relapse after 8 months of maintenance. Prior to suggesting any future strategies, this time factor should be considered.

If clients feel that they are not ready to make another attempt at this time, then this decision should be supported. As long as clients are encouraged to return should they change their minds, then this is a perfectly acceptable outcome. If, however, the client wishes to continue with the change process then some of the behavioural strategies discussed in the previous two chapters will be required again. As with the first attempt at change though, good planning is required. It should be conveyed to the client that the problem(s) that led to the relapse can be managed. As the preparation stage suggested, the following should be discussed prior to arriving at an action plan.

- Detailed discussion of the problem or high risk situation.
- Menu of coping strategies.
- Selection of option client thinks is best at this time.
- Plan to implement the option.

Encouraging clients to see the options as an opportunity to experiment and to find out what works best for them is important. None of the high risk situations are insurmountable, although some will need more experimentation than others.

In summary, when clients have slipped or relapsed they will re-use the processes of self-reevaluation and self-liberation. They may see themselves as weak, hopeless and more attached to the old behaviour than they first thought. They will also recognise that they have had some success at behaviour change. It is the practitioner's task to help clients see the causes of their slips or relapses as controllable external factors that are not proof of any inherent weakness. In addition, the practitioner can help clients renew their commitment to change and remind themselves of their belief that change is possible.

Chapter 14
Weight Management

Many people seeking advice on changing eating and exercise behaviours do so specifically because they wish to lose weight. This chapter will focus on the special considerations of weight control that are different for the general eating and exercise strategies outlined so far in this book.

Despite more and more people attempting to lose weight, the number of overweight and obese people in the population is growing and now over half of the adult population in the UK has a body mass index (BMI) of 25 or more (Health Survey for England 1993). It is commonly stated that 95% of attempts to lose weight are unsuccessful in the long term (Campbell 1995). In other words, the majority of people who attempt to lose weight usually return to their original weight and some cases even gain weight. Practitioners should be realistic, therefore, about the likely success rate of working with overweight and obese clients. This does not mean being resigned to the fact that weight loss is not possible, but recognising that it requires sustained hard work, which a lot of clients are not ready to undertake. People are always looking for a quick and easy way to lose weight.

Many of the weight loss programmes being marketed to those wishing to lose weight have no evidence of their efficacy and may be unsafe. In an attempt to protect the consumer from false advertising claims and to establish an acceptable standard of healthcare in weight loss programmes, a number of organisations have drawn up guidelines for audit weight loss programmes (American College of Sports Medicine 1983, Task Force to Establish Weight Loss Guidelines 1990). The main points which emerge from them all are listed below.

● Clients should be screened and the level of health risk established before the programme is started.

- Treatment plans should be individualised.
- The staff who administer the programmes should be appropriately trained.
- A reasonable weight goal should be established with consideration given to personal and family history. It should not be based solely on height weight charts.
- The diet should include foods acceptable to the dieter in terms of sociocultural background, usual habits, taste, costs and ease of acquisition and preparation.
- The minimum calorie intake should be 1200 kcals/day. (Only in extreme cases with close medical supervision, should intakes fall below this level.)
- Average weight loss should not exceed 2 lb (1 kg) per week.
- The diet should be nutritionally balanced.
- The diet should include an exercise programme that promotes a daily caloric expenditure of 300 or more kcal.
- Behaviour modification techniques should be included.
- Appetite suppressant drugs should be avoided.
- Weight maintenance should be as much a priority as weight loss.
- The programme should be sustainable in the long term.

It is beyond the scope of this book to review all of the weight control literature and readers are recommended to familiarise themselves with the facts from a comprehensive text such as *Eating Disorders and Obesity* (Brownell & Fairburn 1995).

As described in Chapter 2 there are undoubted health risks associated with obesity (BMI over 30), though the extent of the risks of carrying a less excess weight (overweight, BMI 25–29.9) are less clear cut. The health risks on which national targets are set are in respect of physical disease such as coronary heart disease and diabetes. Some authors have suggested, however, that the psychosocial damage caused by being overweight and obese carries additional risks to mental health, contributes to overall health and is often overlooked.

There is also some debate about the psychological damage which can be the result of repeated unsuccessful attempts to 'diet' and yo-yo dieting by those who are chronically obese. There is an argument that perhaps more harm than good results in psychosocial terms when people try to lose weight but do not succeed (Wooley & Garner 1991, Brownell & Rodin 1994). Their weight remains high and their mental health is worse because they think of themselves as having failed and being weak and worthless. This applies not only to obese people, who are more likely to have a long history of weight loss attempts, but also to those who are marginally overweight or actually at the upper end of the healthy weight range for their height and keep trying to lose weight.

Health and fitness professionals should be mindful of this potential scenario and work with the client towards realistic outcomes, as described earlier. By developing the skills and using the approaches described throughout this book your counselling and support should not be counterproductive. Remember that weight stability, that is prevention of further weight gain, can be seen as a positive outcome.

Decisions about when to raise the issue and attempt to motivate clients towards changing their weight can clearly be made on health grounds alone. Often clients will raise the issue themselves, particularly in the fitness setting. When discussing people's weight and whether or not they wish to consider trying to lose weight, consideration should be given both to the health risks of not reducing their weight and also to some of the difficulties associated with losing weight. Being clear-cut about risk can be quite difficult and there remains some debate as to when weight starts to be a health risk.

The cut-off points used for the BMI ranges have been developed from curves which show the association of body weight with healthy risk, measured using morbidity (rate of disease) and mortality (rate of death) statistics. The risk to health starts to increase at a BMI of around 25, which is why this figure is suggested as the upper limit for good health. The curve becomes more steep at a BMI of around 28 and some have suggested that this is the point at which risk to health is really becoming problematic. The argument for choosing the BMI limit of 25 for good health is that it is better to try to prevent people getting to the BMI of 28, rather than waiting until they get there and then trying to help them prevent further weight gain, or reduce weight. A BMI of 30 or more, that is overt obesity, is a clear indicator for practitioners to raise the issue.

Someone who is overweight though not obese, but has associated risk factors for disease such as high blood pressure, diabetes, high blood cholesterol levels or physical inactivity has an overall risk which is approaching that of an obese person, so should be managed accordingly.

An additional consideration when assessing the health risk of carrying excess weight is the distribution of the fat. There is an increasingly convincing body of evidence showing that central fat deposition (apple shaped fatness) poses a great risk to health than peripheral fat deposition (pear shaped fatness). That is, someone who carries most of their excess fat around the stomach and waist is more at risk of disease than a person who has excess fat on the hips and thighs and has a trim waist. This can be measured by calculating the 'waist-hip ratio' (WHR); where the figure exceeds one, meaning the waist measurement (the smallest circumference of the torso) is greater than the hip measurement (the largest circumference around the hips and buttocks), the person has central adiposity and is therefore at greater health risk.

In addition to being aware of the health risks described above, clients wishing to modify their weight should first understand the energy balance equation. That is, that body mass remains constant when caloric intake equals caloric expenditure as shown in Figure 14.1. A person's body weight mainly reflects the balance between these two things. That is, firstly the energy taken in, in the form of food, and secondly the energy expended. Energy expended includes the basal metabolic rate (BMR – the minimum energy required for the body to perform its normal functions while

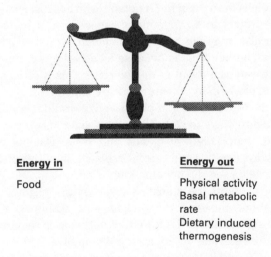

Energy in

Food

Energy out

Physical activity
Basal metabolic
rate
Dietary induced
thermogenesis

When energy in = energy out, body weight is stable.

Figure 14.1   The energy balance equation.

awake), the level of physical activity and the energy expended from eating, known as dietary induced thermogenesis (DIT).

BMR accounts for the largest proportion of energy expenditure, approximately 60–65%, with DIT being the smallest at around 5%. The remaining 30–35% can be expended through physical activity (Katch & McArdle 1993). This proportion can be lower or higher depending on how physically active a person is.

Although the energy expended through BMR and DIT varies within individuals, people have no voluntary control over this variation. Increasing activity levels is the only possible strategy for increasing overall energy expenditure. A tiny minority of people have metabolic and/or hormonal abnormalities which will influence their weight, but for the majority, weight reflects the amount of food we eat and how much physical activity we take. When our energy expenditure is greater than our energy intake we are said to be in a negative energy balance leading to a decrease in body mass. When energy expenditure is less than energy intake, we are in positive energy balance leading to an increase in body mass. When energy expenditure equals energy intake, energy is balanced and body mass is stable. An easy way to remember this is with the rhyme 'More in than out – you're stout. More out than in – you're thin'.

Body weight is also influenced by body composition because muscle weighs more than fat. A person who has lost some body fat through a weight loss programme, especially if it includes resistance exercise, may not have lost as much overall weight as they would have hoped. This is because lean tissue (i.e. muscle) may have increased as a result of the exercise. This is often a cause of concern expressed by clients who are fixated on the weighing scales as the best indicator of progress. We would recommend that one of the best ways to assess healthy weight loss is the tightness of clothes, especially waistbands and belts! Gaining muscle is almost always positive and careful explanation of this at the outset will help clients see the benefits more clearly.

Bearing in mind the statistics given at the beginning of this chapter about unsuccessful weight loss attempts, it is very important for clients to think hard about what is required to lose weight before starting out on a programme of weight control. The practitioner's role is to help the client progress logically throughout each of the stages of change. So, by the time they have reached a decision to try to take more exercise and/or eat more healthily, they have thought it through and have a well prepared plan of action. As mentioned earlier, moving too rapidly to the action stage increases the likelihood of relapse because the barriers have not been considered and a realistic way of working towards the goal, which suits the individual, has not been prepared.

Most clients considering losing weight are equally motivated by two conflicting goals. On the one hand they are very motivated to lose weight and yet on the other they are very motivated to maintain their current eating and exercising habits. In other words, they are very ready to be at a lower weight but not ready at all to alter their eating and exercise behaviour to achieve this end. This can become confusing and misleading when clients present themselves for help to lose weight. It is easy to be fooled into thinking that clients are highly motivated and are ready for action when in fact they can be in precontemplation or contemplation. To avoid this confusion, it is important to make the distinction between a desired outcome and the changes in behaviour(s) required to achieve that outcome. For example, 'I can see that you are very keen to lose weight. I wonder if you have given any thought to what aspects of your lifestyle might need to change in order to achieve that'.

This kind of open-ended question can help focus clients' minds on the behaviours that influence the outcome they are looking for. It is similar to clients who turn up at a health club and state that they want to get fit. Fitness is a physiological outcome that can be derived from changes in physical activity, a behaviour. So the first task in helping a client lose weight can often be showing them the relationship between a physical measure, such as body mass, and their behaviour, i.e. eating and exercise. Having done this, the client can see that changing both eating and exercise behaviours is required in order to lose weight. The next step is to establish how ready the client is to change either of the behaviours, which will reflect how motivated they are to lose weight. Some clients may be ready to change one behaviour more than the other. For this reason, it is important to treat them separately. So while you may be able to negotiate a plan for changing eating behaviour, you may need to spend more time on motivational strategies for exercise behaviour.

When the stage of change for each behaviour has been established, the appropriate processes of change for that stage should be used (see previous chapters). As the client will be keen to start making progress towards their goal of losing weight, it may be sensible to do more work with the behaviour that they are more ready to change. If practitioners spend a lot of time initially trying to motivate the client to think about changing their eating behaviour, when they are already in the preparation stage for exercise behaviour, they are likely to become irritated and resistant. Not that this means that they should completely abandon the other behaviour. It is probably easier to re-introduce the second behaviour when clients are frustrated by the slow rate of progress they are making by just modifying one behaviour.

When clients are showing commitment to change and are ready to consider options for change, their decision making may be influenced by the rate of weight change they are expecting or hoping for. The following explanation should help make this point clear.

Each pound of 0.45 kg of body fat contains approximately 3500 kcals. To lose weight at a rate of 1 lb a week therefore, a daily negative energy balance of 500 kcal would need to be established. If this was done by only modifying the amount of physical activity taken each day, it would mean taking 1 hour of moderately vigorous exercise for all of the 7 days in the week. For the vast majority of people this represents a significant change in exercise behaviour and is unrealistic. It would be equally difficult to create this deficit by only changing eating behaviour. A 500 kcal/day reduction in food intake would represent about a 28% reduction in total calorie intake for women and about a 22% reduction for men (based on average energy input). Combining changes in eating and exercise, however, means that the same negative energy balance can be obtained, but with more moderate, sustainable changes in behaviour. Using the examples given above, the same gain could be achieved by doing exercise on only 3 or 4 days of the week, combined with a dietary restriction of about 10–15% of energy intake per day.

It is important to show clients this relationship between changes in their behaviour and the extent of the changes in their weight. If they have unrealistic expectations about how much weight they will lose each week or month, they are likely to become frustrated very early on. This may be one of the main reasons why so many clients return to their old eating and exercise patterns.

The literature on the rate of weight loss and weight maintenance suggests that people do better in the long term when average

weight lost does not exceed 2 lb per week (Drewnowski 199[
is not surprising when one considers the degree of cha
behaviour required just to lose 1 lb/week. Clients wanting t
weight more quickly than this should be made aware of the u111-
culties and the limitations. Even if they are committed enough to
put in the hard effort required to achieve weight loss quickly (e.g.
for an important occasion such as a family wedding or a holiday)
they should be offered information about the dangers of losing
weight quickly. This is along the theme that 'dieting makes you fat'.
It is possible that rapid weight loss is a result of loss of body muscle
and water as well as fat. Therefore, the final goal weight may be
achieved but the weight almost inevitably will gradually creep back
on. The weight gained is likely to have a higher proportion of fat
than that lost because it is regained more gradually. The result is
that the person may be back at the original weight (before the
weight loss attempt) according to the weighing scales, but the
proportion of body fat is actually higher. This can reduce metabolic
rate, making subsequent weight loss attempts even more difficult.

Having established a reasonable weight goal with clients within a
reasonable time frame, consideration should be given to more
specific change options for eating and exercise. These may differ
slightly from the options already discussed in earlier chapters.

Exercise

For the purpose of weight loss, exercise can be viewed as energy
expenditure. Therefore, any energy expenditure greater than that
which is currently being expended will contribute to weight loss. A
calorie expended is a calorie expended. This means that clients
have a lot more flexibility over the type of exercise they choose to
take up. The energy expended from physical activity is influenced
by the frequency, duration and intensity. It is not important that
people exercise for a minimum duration, such as 30 minutes, or a
minimum intensity such as moderate. Any activity helps to boost
energy expenditure and the activity which the client most enjoys is
more likely to be sustained.

For people who are overweight and obese, it is important to
acknowledge that their life experience of sport and activity may
have been very negative. If they were overweight as a child, it is
possible that they will have been teased and ridiculed in physical

activity sessions at school, will not have been 'good' at any sport and will not have developed any skills which might have increased their confidence about exercising. Likewise, overweight adults may have felt self-conscious about wearing the type of clothes which are required for exercising (swimming costumes, shorts), or may have felt too immobile or clumsy to participate actively in any form of recreation or leisure pursuits. In essence, the practitioners task is to help them feel more confident and optimistic about their participation and enjoyment in any form of activity, however small.

When considering advice for overweight and obese people about exercise, safety should be considered. Many overweight clients find some types of exercise particularly uncomfortable. In general, exercises that involve high impact such as jogging or high impact aerobic classes should be avoided. Weight bearing exercises such as cycling and swimming are normally much better tolerated by overweight people and are less stressful on knee and hip joints. Overweight clients tend to have a lower tolerance for exercise than people who are within the healthy weight range, so they will tend to become fatigued more quickly. Exercise carried out more frequently, but at a lower intensity and shorter duration, is therefore normally preferred by clients who are overweight or obese.

Clients will be encouraged by the knowledge that they can accumulate their exercise in small bouts throughout the day, such as 10 minutes at a time, all of which will contribute to an increased energy expenditure. It has been recommended that people trying to lose weight should aim towards accumulating 1000 kcals per week of extra energy expenditure (ACSM 1995). This is equivalent to approximately 2 miles of walking on 5 days of the week.

As well as increasing total energy expenditure, exercise combined with food restriction enhances fat loss and minimises losses of lean tissue (Hill *et al.* 1994). Perhaps one of the most important reasons for including exercise in a weight loss attempt is that it is one of the few factors correlated with the maintenance of a lower body weight. In other words, subjects who exercise during weight loss seem to do better at weight maintenance than those who do not exercise.

Eating

For the purposes of weight loss, eating can be viewed as energy intake. Therefore, any energy intake less than that which is currently being eaten will contribute to weight loss. A calorie less is a calorie less but the nutritional quality of what is eaten is also important for overall health. A chocolate bar and a bag of chips, in total would provide less than 1000 calories, but nutritionally speaking would represent a disastrous daily eating plan. The food groups approach, described in Chapter 10, describes how best to achieve nutritional balance in the diet. The message is clear and simple: plenty of 'fruit and vegetables' and 'bread, other cereals and potatoes', moderate amounts of 'milk and dairy' and 'meat, fish and alternative' foods and small and/or infrequent amounts of food from the 'fatty and sugary foods' group. People wanting to reduce their overall energy intake should be especially vigilant to ensure they are eating:

● enough 'fruit and vegetables' and 'bread, cereals and potato' (without added fat whenever possible);
● fewer portions of foods from the 'fatty and sugary' group; and
● low fat choices from the 'milk and dairy' and 'meat, fish and alternative' groups.

The minimum in the range of portion sizes given in the National Food Guide in Figure 10.1 are as low as anyone should go, including people who are trying to lose weight. The portions would provide about 1200 kcal and this is the recommended minimum energy intake in adults. Clients who wish to eat fewer calories, or claim they already are, will be hindering, not helping their weight loss attempt. A daily diet providing less than 1200 calories may well be nutritionally incomplete and not sufficiently filling to be sustainable in the long term. Maintaining such intakes for even a few days will probably result in feelings of hunger, weakness, tiredness and unwillingness to take exercise, all of which defeat the whole object of the eating plan.

Further detail about some dietary regimes which are not recommended are given in Chapter 10. Fuller explanations about the physiology and biochemistry of eating for weight loss are given in a text recommended previously. (Brownell & Fairburn 1995).

Summary

Working with weight control is not the same as working with eating or exercise as individual behaviours. When considering controlling their weight, clients have multiple behaviours to consider for change. The practitioner's task is to help clients decide which behaviour(s), if any, they wish to tackle first. Although there are some technical differences in the eating and exercise options when applied to weight control, the processes of change are the same once the behaviour for change has been identified.

References

Ahmed F.E. (1992) Effect of nutrition on the health of the elderly. *Journal of the American Dietetic Association*, **92**(9), 1102–1108.

Allied Dunbar (1992) *Allied Dunbar National Fitness Survey. Main Findings.* Sports Council and Health Education Authority, London.

American College of Sports Medicine (1983) Proper and improper weight loss programmes. *Medicine, Science, Sports and Exercise*, **15**, ix–xiii.

American College of Sports Medicine (1990) The recommended quantity and quality of exercise for developing and maintaining cardiorespiratory and muscular fitness in healthy adults. *Medicine, Science, Sports and Exercise*, **22**, 265–274.

American College of Sports Medicine (1995) *Guidelines for Exercise Testing and Prescription*, 5th edn. Lea & Febiger, Philadelphia.

Ammerman A.S., DeVellis B.M., Haines P.S. *et al.* (1992) Nutrition education for cardiovascular disease prevention among low income populations: description and pilot evaluation of a physician-based model. *Patient Education and Counselling*, **19**, 5–18.

Baron J.A., Gleason R., Crowe B. & Mann J.I. (1990) Preliminary trial of the effect of general practice based nutritional advice. *British Journal of General Practitioners*, **40**, 137–141.

Berlin J.A. & Colditz G.A. (1990) A meta-analysis of physical activity in the prevention of coronary heart disease. *American Journal of Epidemiology*, **132**, 639–646.

Beresford S.A., Farmer E.M., Feingold I. *et al.* (1992) Evaluation of a self-help dietary intervention in a primary care setting. *American Journal of Public Health*, **82**, 79–94.

Biddle S., Fox K. & Edmunds L. (1994) *Physical Activity Promotion in Primary Health Care in England.* Health Education Authority, London.

Bingham S. (1991) Dietary aspects of a health strategy for England. The Health of the Nation: responses. *British Medical Journal*, **303**, 353–355.

Blair S.N. *et al.* (1985) Assessment of habitual physical activity by a seven-day recall in a community survey and controlled experiments. *American Journal of Epidemiology*, **122**, 794–804.

Blair S.N. *et al.* (1989) Physical fitness and all-cause mortality. A prospective study of healthy men and woman. *Journal of the American Medical Association*, **262**, 2395–2401.

Blair S.N., Kohl H.W. & Gordon N.F. (1992) How much physical activity is enough? *Annual Review of Public Health*, **13**, 99–126.

Bouchard C., Shephard R.J. & Stephens T. (1994) *Physical Activity, Fitness and Health: International Proceedings and Consensus Statement 1992*. Human Kinetics Publishers, Champaign, Illinois.

Brownell K.D. & Rodin J. (1994) The dieting maelstrom. Is it possible and advisable to lose weight? *American Psychologist*, **49**, 781–791.

Brownell K.D. & Fairburn C.G. (1995) *Eating Disorders and Obesity: A Comprehensive Handbook*. The Guildford Press, New York.

Cade J. & O'Connell (1992) Management of weight problems and obesity: knowledge, attitudes and current practice of general practitioners. *British Journal of General Practice*, **41**, 147–150.

Campbell K. (1995) *Obesity in Primary Health Care: A Literature Review*. Health Education Authority, London.

Cousins J.H., Rubovits D.S., Dunn J.K. *et al.* (1992) Family versus individually oriented intervention for weight loss in Mexican American women. *Public Health Report*, **107**, 549–555.

Dallongville J., Leboeuf N., Blais C. *et al.* (1994) Short-term response to dietary counselling of hyperlipdaemic outpatients of a lipid clinic. *Journal of the American Dietetic Association*, **94**, 616–621.

Denke M.A. & Grundy S.M. (1994) Individual responses to a cholesterol-lowering diet in 50 men with moderate hypercholesterolaemia. *Archives of Internal Medicine*, **154**, 317–325.

Department of Health and Social Security (1984) *Diet and Cardiovascular Disease: Report of the Panel on Diet in Relation to Cardiovascular Disease, Committee on Medical Aspects of Food Policy. Report on Health and Social Subjects No. 28*. HMSO, London.

Department of Health (1991) *Dietary Reference Values for Food Energy and Nutrients for the United Kingdom. Report on Health and Social Subjects No. 41*. HMSO, London.

Department of Health (1992) *The Health of the Nation. A Strategy for Health for England*. DoH, London.

Department of Health (1994a) *Nutritional Aspects of Cardiovascular Disease. A Report of the Cardiovascular Review Group of the Committee on Medical Aspects of Food Policy. Report on Health and Social Subjects No. 46*. HMSO, London.

Department of Health (1994b) *Eat Well. An Action Plan from the Nutrition Task Force to Achieve the Health of the Nation Targets on Diet and Nutrition*. DoH, London.

Dishman R.K. & Sallis J.F. (1994) Determinants and interventions for physical activity and exercise. In *Physical Activity, Fitness and Health: International Proceedings and Consensus Statement 1992* (eds Bouchard C., Shephard R.J. & Stephens T.), pp. 214–238. Human Kinetics Publishers, Champaign, Illinois.

Drewnowski A. (1995) Standards for the treatment of obesity. In *Eating Disorders and Obesity: A Comprehensive Handbook* (eds Brownell K.D. & Fairburn C.G.). Human Kinetics Publishers, Champaign, Illinois.

Egan G. (1994) *The Skilled Helper. A Problem-Management Approach to Helping*, 5th edn. Brooks/Cole, Pacific Grove, California.

Fagard R.H. & Tipton C.M. (1994) Physical activity, fitness and hypertension. In *Physical Activity, Fitness and Health: International Proceedings and Consensus Statement 1992* (eds Bouchard C., Shephard R.J. & Stephens T.), pp. 633–655. Human Kinetics Publishers, Champaign, Illinois.

Family Heart Study Group (1994) Randomised control trial evaluating cardiovascular screening and intervention in general practice: principal results of the British family heart study. *British Medical Journal*, **308**, 313–320.

Francis J., Roche M. & Mant D. 1989) Would primary health care workers give appropriate dietary advice after cholesterol screening? *British Medical Journal*, **298**, 1620–1622.

Gatenby S.J., Hunt P. & Rayner M. (1995) The National Food Guide: development of dietetic and nutritional characteristics. *Journal of Human Nutrition and Dietetics*, **8**(5), 47–58.

Geiger C.J., Wyse B.W., Parent C.R.M. & Hansen R.G. (1991) Review of nutrition labelling formats. *Journal of the American Dietetic Association*, **91**, 808–815.

Gemson D.H., Sloan R.P., Messeri P. *et al.* (1990) A public health model for cardiovascular risk reduction. Impact of cholesterol screening with brief non-physician counselling. *Archives of Internal Medicine*, **150**, 985–989.

Geppert J. & Splett P.L. (1991) Summary document of nutrition interventions in obesity. *Journal of the American Dietetic Association Supplement*, S31–35.

Glanz K. (1985) Nutrition education for risk factor reduction and patient education: a review. *Preventive Medicine*, **14**, 725–752.

Glanz K. & Eriksen M. (1993) Individual and community models for dietary behaviour change. *Journal of Nutrition Education*, **25**(2), 80–86.

Gregory J.K., Foster K., Tyler H. & Wiseman M. (1990) *The dietary and nutritional survey of British adults*. HMSO, London.

Greene G.W., Rossi S.R., Richards-Reed G., Willey C. & Prochaska J.O. (1994) Stages of change for reducing dietary fat to 30% of energy or less. *Journal of the American Dietetic Association*, **94**(10), 1105–1110.

Hany S., Greminger P., Angermeier M. *et al.* (1990) Effect of a follow-up action in diet instruction. *Schweiz Rundsc. Med. Prax*, **79**, 719–725.

Health Education Authority (1993) *Nutrition Interventions in Primary Care – A Literature Review. A Nutrition Briefing Paper.* HEA, London.

Heller R.F., Elliot H., Bray A.E. & Alabaster M. (1989) Reducing blood cholesterol levels in patients with peripheral disease: dietitian or fact sheet? *Medical Journal of Australia*, **151**, 566–568.

Hill J.O., Drougas H.J. & Peters J.C. (1994) Physical activity, fitness and moderate obesity. In *Physical Activity, Fitness and Health: International Proceedings and Consensus Statement 1992* (eds Bouchard C., Shephard R.J. & Stephens T.), pp. 684–695. Human Kinetics Publishers, Champaign, Illinois.

Hillsdon M., Thorogood M., Anstiss T. & Morris J. (1995) Randomised controlled trials of physical activity promotion in free living adults: a review. *Journal of Epidemiology and Community Health*, **49**, 448–453.

Hunt P. (1992) Nutrition communication – the community view. In *Getting the Message Across – Nutrition and Communication* (ed. Butriss J.). National Dairy Council, London.

Hunt P. (1995a) Dietary counselling: theory and practice. *Journal of the Institute of Health Education*, **33**(1), 4–8.

Hunt P., Gatenby S.J. & Rayner M. (1995b) A national food guide for the UK? Background and development. *Journal of Human Nutrition and Dietetics*, **8**(5), 39–46.

Hunt P. Gatenby S.J. & Rayner M. (1995c) The format for the National Food Guide; performance and preference studies. *Journal of Human Nutrition and Dietetics*, **8**(5), 59–75.

Hunt P. (1995d) Development and evaluation of the Changing What You Eat resources for primary care. *Health Education Journal*, **54**, 405–414.

Imperial Cancer Research Fund OXCHECK Study Group (1994) Effectiveness of health checks conducted by nurses in primary care: results of the OXCHECK study after one year. *British Medical Journal*, **308**, 308–312.

Iso H., Konishi M., Terao A. *et al.* (1991) A community based education program for serum cholesterol reduction in urban hypercholesterolaemic persons – comparisons of intensive and usual education groups. *Nippon. Koshu. Eisei. Zasshi*, **66**, 751–761.

Katch F.I. & McArdle W.D. (1993) *Introduction to Exercise, Nutrition and Health* 4th edn. Lea & Febiger, Philadelphia.

Kelly R.B., Zyzanksi S.J. & Alemagno S.A. (1991) Prediction of motivation and behaviour change following health promotion: role of health beliefs, social support and self-efficacy. *Social Science and Medicine*, **32**, 311–320.

Keuhl K.S., Cockerham J.T., Hotchings M. *et al.* (1994) Effective control of hypercholesterolaemia in children with dietary interventions based in pediatric practice. *Preventive Medicine*, **22**, 154–166.

Kumar N.B., Bostow D.E., Schapira D.V. *et al.* (1993) Efficacy of inter-active, automated programmed instruction in nutrition education for cancer prevention. *Journal of Cancer Education*, **8**, 203–211.

Kupka Schutt L. & Mitchell M.E. (1992) Positive effect of a nutrition instruction model on the dietary behaviour of a selected group of elderly. *Journal of Nutrition for the Elderly*, **12**, 29–53.

Kyle A. (1993). Are practice nurses an effective means of delivering dietary advice as part of health promotion in primary health care? Evaluation of practice nurse training in Somerset. *Journal of Human Nutrition and Dietetics*, **6**, 149–162.

Law M.R., Wald N.J., Thompson S.G. (1994). By how much and how quickly does reduction in serum cholesterol concentration lower risk of ischaemic heart disease? *British Medical Journal*, **308**, 367–372.

Lefebvre R.C., Lasater T.M. Carelton R.A., Peterson G. (1987). Theory and delivery of healthy promoting in the community: The Pawtucket Heart Health Programme. *Preventive Medicine*, **16**, 80–95.

Longfield J., Rayner M. & Roe L. (1995) *Dietary Counselling – A Literature Review. Internal Report for the Health Education Authority's Primary Care Unit, Oxford.*

Marlatt G.A. & Gordon J.R. (1985) *Relapse Prevention: Maintenance Strategies in the Treatment of Addictive Behaviours.* The Guildford Press, New York.

McCluney J. (1988) *Answering back: Public Views on Food and Health Information.* Horton, Bradford.

McGowan M.P., Joffe A., Duggan A.K. & McCay P.S. (1994) Intervention in hypercholesterolaemic college students: a pilot study. *Journal of Adolescent Health*, **15**, 155–162.

Miller W. (1983) Motivational interviewing with problem drinkers. *Behavioural Psychotherapy*, **11**, 147–172.

Miller W.R. & Rollnick S. (1991) *Motivational Interviewing: Preparing People to Change Addictive Behaviour.* The Guildford Press, New York.

Mullen P.D., Mains D.A. & Velez R. (1992) A meta-analysis of controlled trials of cardiac patient education. *Patient Education and Counselling*, **19**, 143–162.

Murray D.M., Kurth C., Mullis R. & Jeffery R.W. (1990) Cholesterol reduction through low intensity interventions: results from the Minnesota Heart Health Programme. *Preventive Medicine*, **19**, 181–189.

Murray S., Narayan V., Mitchell M. & Wite H. (1993) Study of dietetic knowledge among members of the primary health care team. *British Journal of General Practice*, **43**, 229–231.

Najavits L.M. & Weiss R.D. (1994) Variations in therapist effectiveness in the treatment of patients with substance use disorders: an empirical review. *Addiction*, **89**, 679–688.

National Dairy Council (1992) Food and health – what does Britain think? NDC, London.

Neale A.V. (1991) Behavioural contracting as a tool to help patients achieve better health. *Family Practice*, **8**, 336–342.

Office of Population and Census Surveys (1994) *National Food Survey*. HMSO, London.

Office of Population and Census Surveys (1994) *Health Survey for England 1992*. HMSO, London.

Office of Population and Census Surveys (1995) *Health Survey for England 1993*. HMSO, London.

O'Connell D. & Velicer W. (1988) A decisional balance measure and the stages of change model for weight loss. *The International Journal of Addictions*, **23**(7), 729–750.

Ornish D., Brown S.E., Scherwitz *et al.* (1990) Can lifestyle changes reverse coronary heart disease? *Lancet*, **336**, 129–33.

Pate R.R., Pratt M., Blair S.N., Haskell W.L., Macera C.A., Bouchard C. *et al.* (1995) Physical activity and public health A recommendation from the Centres for Disease Control and Prevention and the American College of Sports Medicine. *Journal of the American Medical Association*, **273**, 402–407.

Pooling Project Research Group (1978) Relationship of blood pressure, serum cholesterol, smoking habit, relative weight and ECG abnormalities to incidence of major coronary events: final report of the pooling project. *Journal of Chronic Disease*, **31**, 202–306.

Powell K.E., Thompson P.D., Caspersen C.J. & Kendrick J.S. (1987) Physical activity and the incidence of coronary heart disease. *Annual Review of Public Health*, **8**, 253–287.

Prochaska J.O. & DiClemente C.C. (1983) Stages and processes of self-change of smoking: toward an integrative model of change. *Journal of Consulting and Clinical Psychology*, **51**, 390–395.

Prochaska J.O. & DiClemente C.C. (1984) *The Transtheoretical Approach: Crossing the Traditional Boundaries of Therapy*. Dow-Jones/Irwin, Homewood, Illinois.

Prochaska J.O. (1994) Strong and weak principles for progressing from precontemplation to action on the basis of twelve problem behaviours. *Health Psychology*, **13**, 47–51.

Prochaska J.O., Velicer W.F., Rossi J.S., Goldstein M.G., Marcus B.H., Rakowkski W. *et al.* (1994) Stages of change and decisional balance for 12 problem behaviours. *Health Psychology*, **13**, 39–46.

Puska P., Salonen J.T. Nissinen A. *et al.* (1983) Change in risk factors for coronary heart disease during 10 years of a community intervention programme (North Karelia Project). *British Medical Journal,* **287,** 1840–1844.

Quaglietti S. & Froelicher V.F. (1994) Physical activity, and cardiac rehabilitation for patients with coronary heart disease. In *Physical Activity, Fitness and Health: International Proceedings and Consensus Statement 1992* (eds Bouchard C., Shephard R.J. & Stephens T.), pp. 591–608. Human Kinetics Publishers, Champaign, Illinois.

Ramsay L.E., Yeo W.W. & Jackson P.R. (1991) Dietary reduction in serum cholesterol concentration; time to think again. *British Medical Journal,* **303,** 953–957.

Roach R.R., Pichert J.W., Stetson B.A. *et al.* (1992) Improving dietitian's teaching skills. *Journal of the American Dietetic Association,* **92,** 1466–1470.

Roe L., Strong C., Whiteside C. *et al.* (1994) Dietary intervention in primary care: validation of the DINE method for diet assessment. *Family Practice,* **11,** 375–381.

Rollnick S., Heather N. & Bell A. (1992) Negotiating behaviour change in medical settings: the development of brief motivational interviewing. *Journal of Mental Health,* **1,** 25–37.

Royal College of General Practitioners (1995) *Morbidity Statistics from General Pactice. Fourth National Study. 1991–2.* OPCS, London.

Sheiham A.M., Marmot M., Taylor B. & Brown A. (1990) In *British Social Attitudes Survey Report. 7th Report* (eds Jowell R., Witherspoon S. & Brook L.). SPCR, London.

Stefanick M.L. & Wood P.D. (1994) Physical activity, lipid and lipoprotein metabolism and lipid transport. In *Physical Activity, Fitness and Health: International Proceedings and Consensus Statement 1992* (eds Bouchard C., Shephard R.J. & Stephens T.), pp. 417–431. Human Kinetics Publishers, Champaign, Illinois.

Stott N.C.H. & Pill R.M. (1990) 'Advise Yes, Dictate No'. Subjects' views on health promotion in the consultation. *Family Practice,* **7,** 125–131.

Task Force to Establish Weight Loss Guidelines (1990) *Toward Safe Weight Loss: Recommendations for Adult Weight Loss Programmes in Michigan.* Michigan Department of Public Health, Lansing.

Thomas J. (1991) *Review of Approaches to Nutrition Education and their Effectiveness.* Internal Health Education Authority Report. HEA, London.

Thomas J. (1994) New approaches to achieving dietary change. *Current Opinion in Lipidology,* **5,** 36–41.

Truswell A.S. (1994) Review of dietary intervention studies: effect on coronary events and on total mortality. *Australian and New Zealand Journal of Medicine,* **24,** 908–106.

Vickery C.E. & Hodges P.A.M. (1986) Counselling strategies for dietary management; expanded possibilities for effective behaviour change. *Journal of American Dietetic Association*, **86**, 924–928.

Wallace P., Cutler S. & Haines A. (1988) Perceptions of weight problems and dietary patterns among general practice patients. *Health Education Journal*, **47**, 7–11.

World Health Organisation Study Group (1990) *Diet, Nutrition and the Prevention of Chronic Diseases. WHO Technical Report Series, 797.* WHO, Copenhagen.

Glossary

Action: one of the stages of change in the transtheoretical model which is the basis of the approach to modifying behaviour in this book. People in the action stage have just started to make changes in their behaviour. This stage lasts 0–6 months.

Adherence: the successful performance of a specific plan of action.

Behaviour: the way in which a person acts, performs or conducts him- or herself. This book is about eating and exercise behaviour. That is, the acts of eating and exercising.

Behaviour modification: attempts to modify a person's eating and exercise behaviour using various processes of change that are matched to a person's stage of change.

Body mass index (BMI): a measure of body weight in relation to height which is related to morbidity and mortality. Weight is measured in kilogrammes and height is in metres. The formula for calculating BMI is weight divided by the square of the height (weight/height^2). The healthy weight range for men and women is BMI 20–24.9. Overweight is defined as BMI 25–29.9 and obesity is defined as BMI 30 +. Underweight is BMI < 20.

Cardiovascular disease (CVD) or event: diseases of the heart and circulatory system including ischaemic heart disease and cerebrovascular disease (i.e. angina, heart attack and stroke), heart murmur and abnormal heart rhythms. CVDs are the leading causes of death in both males and females in the UK.

Client: the consumer of care. The person making changes in their behaviour.

Contemplation: one of the stages of change in the transtheoretical model which is the basis of the approach to modifying behaviour in this book. People in this stage of change are seriously considering a change in behaviour but feel ambivalent about it. They can see the advantages of change but can equally see the disadvantages or difficulties involved in changing.

Counselling: the process of assisting or guiding clients, by a trained person on a professional basis, to resolve difficulties. There are many different styles of counselling based on different theories of human behaviour. It is commonly associated with work involving people with mental health or emotional problems. In this book, counselling refers to a helping relationship where one person (the practitioner) is helping another (the client) towards a healthier lifestyle through negotiation, advice and support. The style is both active and directive, while remaining client centred, as opposed to the style of person-centred counselling, which is completely client led.

Diet: a person's habitual eating pattern. Often inappropriately associated with small amounts of special kinds of food eaten on a short-term basis, suggesting severe restriction and denial.

Eating plan: the way people eat which includes a wide range of foods which are filling and enjoyable.

Exercise: a form of physical activity that is planned, structured and involves repetitive bodily movement (e.g. walking), performed to improve or maintain one or more components of physical fitness. Often undertaken with the intention of regaining, maintaining or improving health.

Food: a nutritious substance taken in to maintain life and growth. A food groups approach is advocated in this book as the theoretical basis for a healthy and nutritionally balanced diet. Although there are strictly no 'good' or 'bad' foods, clearly some foods are better and some worse in terms of health.

Functional benefits: the tangible rewards which directly result from a given activity or behaviour. Eating a lower fat diet can lead to a reduced body weight. Taking regular exercise can mean being able to climb stairs unassisted.

Hypertension: high blood pressure. Increases the risk of developing some CVDs.

Lifestyle: the particular way in which a person lives his or her life. In this book the term relates to health-related behaviours such as eating, exercise, smoking and drinking alcohol.

Maintenance: one of the stages of change in the transtheoretical model which is the basis of the approach to modifying behaviour in this book. People at this stage have successfully adhered to a plan of change for at least 6 months. They are attempting to consolidate changes made so far and avoid a return to the old behaviour.

Nutrients: substances, contained in foods, which provide energy and raw materials for the synthesis and maintenance of living material. Nutrients include protein, carbohydrate, fat, alcohol, vitamins and minerals. All of the different nutrients are required in the correct amounts for good health. The National Food Guide, *The Balance of Good Health*, is a practical way of showing the types and proportions of foods from the different food groups which would make up a nutritionally balanced and complete diet.

Obese: very overweight. A body weight that leads to an increased risk of ill-health and disease. A BMI of 30 +.

Outcome: the result of a specific plan of behaviour.

Overweight: weighing more than a healthy weight for height. A BMI of 25–29.9.

Patient: a person receiving or registered to receive a medical treatment.

Physical activity: any bodily movement produced by skeletal muscles that results in energy expenditure.

Physical fitness: a set of attributes which people have or achieve that relates to their ability to perform physical activity.

Precontemplation: one of the stages of change in the transtheoretical model which is the basis of the approach to modifying behaviour in this book. People in this stage are not considering the possibility of a change in their behaviour, either because they do not wish to, or are not aware of the need for change.

Preparation: one of the stages of change in the transtheoretical model which is the basis of the approach to modifying behaviour in this book. People in this stage have made a commitment to change although they may still be somewhat ambivalent about change. They are considering options for change.

Prescription: literally 'a doctor's instruction for the composition and use of a medicine' or an 'instruction to follow a particular course of action'. Is used inappropriately in eating and exercise as 'dietary prescription' and 'exercise prescription'. Implies that the practitioner is in the position of authority and power, and the client is the passive recipient of the prescription.

Prevention: activities or interventions designed to stop, delay or reduce the risk of ill-health.

Primary care: First-line management of health, which could be in a healthcare setting (e.g. surgery or health centre) or in a non-health setting (e.g. community centre, leisure centre or health club).

Primary prevention: activities targeted at a whole population which aim to influence the overall health status and disease prevalence of the given population, rather than targeting those at high risk or with clinical symptoms of a disease.

Processes of change: techniques and strategies which are used to help people progress through the stages of change. Processes of change should be matched to the appropriate stage of change according to the transtheoretical model of change.

Relapse: a temporary or permanent return to the less desired behaviour. The result of an unsuccessful attempt at action or maintenance, normally leading to a return to one of the earlier stages of change.

Risk factor: behaviours or biological, physiological, social psychological and environmental factors, the presence of which increase the risk of developing a given disease. CVD risk factors include smoking, lack of exercise, high fat diet, elevated cholesterol, hypertension, low fitness, obesity, stress and poverty.

Secondary prevention: activities targeted at those who have been identified as being at risk, or having early symptoms of disease, which aim to reduce the prevalence of the disease.

Termination: the most desirable outcome of any attempt to change behaviour. Characterised by zero temptation to return to the 'old' behaviour and 100% confidence to continue with the 'new' behaviour.

Tertiary prevention: activities targeted at those with existing disease, which aim to reduce suffering, disability and death from the disease.

Transtheoretical model of change: a model of behaviour change developed from observing people attempting to stop smoking on their own. An attempt to integrate diverse systems of psychotherapy into a comprehensive model of change for working with addictive behaviours. Includes the stages and processes of change.

Appendix A

**Self-administered form for assessing eating behaviour.
(Reproduced with kind permission of the Health Education
Authority.)**

WHAT DO YOU EAT?

Name _____ Date _____

1. Who does the food shopping for your home? _____

2. Who cooks? _____

3. What cooking and storage facilities do you have?

    Oven [ ]   Microwave [ ]   Freezer [ ]   None [ ]

    Hob [ ]   Fridge   [ ]   Other   [ ]

4. Do you eat breakfast?   Always [ ] Usually [ ] Rarely [ ] Never [ ]

5. How many main or cooked meals do you tend to eat each day? _____

6. How many light meals do you tend to eat each day? _____
    (This means sandwiches, soup, something on toast, etc.)

7. How many snacks do you tend to eat each day? _____
    (This means biscuits, crisps, chocolate, etc.)

8. How many times each week do you eat meals away from home? _____

9. If you eat away from home, write down the type of foods you eat most often:

    from a shop, sandwich bar or kiosk _____

    in the canteen _____

    in a restaurant _____

    in other people's houses _____

    packed lunches _____

10. Are you on a special diet? Yes [ ] No [ ] Unsure [ ]

    If yes, describe it. _____

How much of the following foods do you eat in a normal day? Remember that these questions are about your *usual* choice of foods. It may help to think of what you ate yesterday. You may eat many of the foods on some days but not on others. Pick an average day. Try to fill in all parts as fully as possible.

11. Bread, cereals and potatoes

_____   breakfast cereals (3 tbs)

_____   bread/toast (slices)

_____   pitta bread (small) or chapati

_____   bread bun or roll ($\frac{1}{2}$)

_____   potatoes/sweet potatoes (egg-sized)

_____   rice, pasta or noodles, cooked (2 tbs)

_____   plaintain/green banana (matchbox sized)

_____   *Total*

12. Fruit and vegetables

_____   vegetables (fresh, tinned or frozen) 2 tbs

_____   salad (small)

_____   fresh fruit (e.g. apple, orange, banana, slice melon)

_____   tinned or stewed fruit (2 tbs)

_____   fruit juice (small glass – 100 ml)

_____   *Total*

13. Milk and dairy foods

milk ($\frac{1}{3}$ pint or 200 ml),

_____   full fat (gold or silver top)

_____   semi-skimmed (red stripey top)

_____   skimmed (blue checked top)

_____   cheese (matchbox sized)

_____   yoghurt/cottage cheese/fromage frais (small pot)

_____   *Total*

14. Meat, fish and alternatives

_____   beef/pork/ham/lamb/liver/kidney/ chicken/fish/3 fish fingers (small amount the size of a pack of playing cards)

_____   eggs (2)

_____   tinned baked beans (3 tbs)

_____   dish based on pulses/lentils or dahl (3 tbs)

_____ nuts and nut products (e.g. peanut butter) (2 tbs)

_____ *Total*

15. Fatty and sugary foods

What kind of spreading fat do you usually use?

_____ butter

_____ low-fat spread

_____ tub/block margarine

_____ unsaturated margarine/spread (e.g. sunflower)

_____ don't use any spread

What kind of cooking oil or fat do you usually use?

_____ lard, dripping or ghee

_____ blended vegetable oil

_____ unsaturated oil (e.g. sunflower)

_____ monounsaturated oil (e.g. olive oil, rapeseed)

How much fat do you eat in a normal day

_____ butter or margarine/spread (teaspoons)

_____ low fat spread (teaspoons)

_____ cooking oil/fat/ghee (teaspoons)

_____ mayonnaise/oily salad dressing (teaspoons)

_____ *Total* (this section only)

16. Fatty and sugary foods (cont.)

_____ sugar, e.g. in drinks (teaspoons)

_____ crisps (small bag)

_____ pork pie/sausage roll (small)

_____ doughnut/Danish pastry

_____ cake or pie (1 slice)

_____ ice cream (scoop)

_____ biscuits (3)

_____ chocolate bar (small)

_____ *Total*

17. Drinks

_____ coffee (cup/mug)

_____ tea (cup/mug)

_____ squash/fizzy drinks (glass/can)

_____ diet/slimline/sugar-free drinks (glass can)

_____ water (glass)

_____ *Total*

18. Alcoholic drinks

_____ beer ($\frac{1}{2}$ pint)

_____ wine (small glass)

_____ spirits (pub measure)

_____ other – liqueur, cocktail (pub measure)

_____ *Total*

19. Other foods

Are there any foods you normally eat that have not been mentioned so far? These might be:

• mixed foods, e.g. pizza, shepherd's pie
• foods which are traditional to you, e.g. lassi, paneer, chevda, homous, baclava
• new foods, e.g. Quorn, yoghurt drink, very low fat spread

If so, list them here:

_____

_____

_____

Appendix B

Physical activity questionnaire

We would like to ask you about your physical activity during the past month. We would like you to recall the actual activities you did during the last month, not a history of what you normally do. We will ask you about *moderate* and *vigorous* activities. We will not be considering light activities such as desk work, slow walking or strolling, light housework, etc.

1 First of all we would like to ask you about moderate activities. *Moderate activities make you feel warm and breath more heavily than usual.* Examples include:
    Brisk walking for pleasure or to work;
    Gardening (weeding, raking, mowing, etc.);
    Cycling for pleasure;
    DIY; and
    Swimming leisurely.
These are just examples and do not include all moderate activities. If the activity you did is not in this list it should at least be as hard as brisk walking to call it moderate.

During the past 4 weeks, on how many days did you do any moderate activities that you performed *continuously for at least 30 minutes?* Number of days of moderate ☐

On average, how long did you spend on each of these moderate activities (record to the nearest 10 minutes)? Number of minutes ☐

2 Next, we would like to ask you about vigorous activities *Vigorous activities make you out of breath and sweaty.* Examples include:
    Jogging/running;
    Competitive sports;
    Swimming lengths continuously;
    Climbing stairs briskly; and
    Fast cycling.
These are just examples and do not include all vigorous activities. If the activity you did is not in this list it should at least be as hard as jogging to call it vigorous.

During the past 4 weeks, on how many days did you do any vigorous activities
that you performed *continuously for at least 20 minutes*.
Number of days of vigorous   [   ]

On average, how long did you spend on each of these vigorous activities (record
to the nearest 10 minutes)?
Number of minutes   [   ]

Appendix C

Pre-activity questionnaire

Please tick all the relevant boxes

		Yes	No
1.	Has your doctor ever said that you have a heart condition *and* that you should only do physical activity recommended by a doctor?	☐	☐
2.	Do you have diabetes mellitus?	☐	☐
3.	Do you feel pain in your chest when you do physical activity?	☐	☐
4.	In the past month, have you had chest pain when you were doing physical activity?	☐	☐
5.	Is your doctor currently prescribing drugs for your blood pressure or heart condition?	☐	☐
6.	Do you lose your balance because of dizziness or do you ever lose consciousness?	☐	☐
7.	Do you have a bone or joint problem that could be made worse by a change in your physical activity?	☐	☐
8.	Do you suffer shortness of breath at rest or with mild exertion?	☐	☐
9.	Do you suffer from unusual fatigue or shortness of breath with usual activities?	☐	☐
10.	Do you get a sharp pain in your lower leg when walking uphill or upstairs which disappears within 1–2 minutes of stopping?	☐	☐
11.	Have either your mother, father or other immediate family had a heart attack or died suddenly prior to the age of 55?	☐	☐
12.	Has your doctor ever said that you have high blood pressure?	☐	☐
13.	Has your doctor said you have raised cholesterol levels?	☐	☐

14. Do you currently smoke cigarettes?   ☐   ☐

15. I do *not* currently exercise on a regular basis (at least 3 times   ☐   ☐
     per week) and/or work in a job that is physically demanding?

16. Do you know of any other reason why you should not do   ☐   ☐
     physical activity?

Refer to flow diagrams below for decisions about safe exercise.

**Physical activity risk stratification (adapted from the American College of
Sports Medicine Guidelines for Exercise Testing and Prescription 1995)**

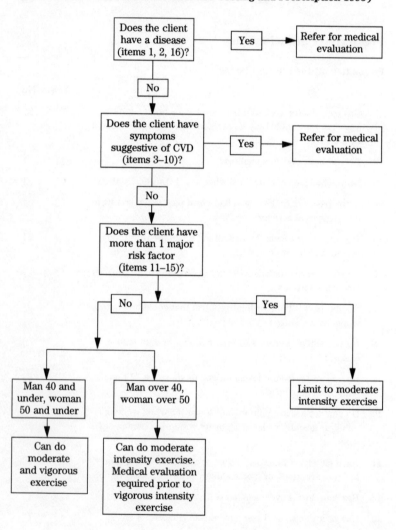

Appendix D

Summary of change plan

The main reasons I want to change are: ....
....
....

The changes I am prepared to make are: ....
....
....

The steps I will take to implement change are: ....
....
....

People who may support me are: ....
....
....

Things that may make change difficult are: ....
....
....

My plans for coping with difficult situations are: ....
....
....

I will know when I've been successful when: ....
....
....

I will reward myself for being successful with: ....
....
....

Appendix E

Self-monitoring diary for one day

Name: _____ Date: _____ Day: _____

Type of food e.g. milk, bread Activity e.g. walking, swimming	Description e.g. semi-skimmed, toast e.g. brisk, leisurely	Amount e.g. 1 mug, 1 tbs e.g. ½ hour, 30 lanes	When e.g. 11 am, lunch time, 9 pm	Where e.g. home, work, cafe, pool	With whom e.g. alone, family, friends	Mood e.g. sad, angry, happy

Index